"The practice of mindfulness is the Buddha's main ingredient in his recipe for lasting peace, happiness and enlightened living. It is only through experiencing this with ourselves that we can heal what ails us, transform ourselves and our relationships, and find true purpose and fulfillment. This wise book provides practical exercises that will help us to develop conscious awareness and inner understanding, and the ways and means to free us from unsatisfying habits, addictions, and unconscious behavior patterns. I recommend it highly."

—Lama Surya Das, author of *Awakening the Buddha Within*

"*Mindful Recovery* combines two hitherto unrelated worlds—that of modern cognitive therapy and Buddhist reflection. The connection makes incredible sense, since Buddhism is not a religion in the traditional sense so much as it is a method for directing one's thoughts and experiences. By centering oneself in one's here-and-now, lived experience, addicts can avoid the infantilism, the regrets, the efforts to seek unrewarding rewards that are the basis for self-destructive behaviors. By reading about and applying these techniques, individuals can work on the internal urges that accompany their addictive problems."

—Stanton Peele, Ph.D., author of *The Truth About Addiction and Recovery* and *The Meaning of Addiction*

"Anyone interested in finding a kind, spiritual guide to recovery that focuses on flexibility rather than the 'one true way' will benefit from this enjoyable and helpful book."

—Maia Szalavitz, coauthor with
Joseph Volpicelli, M.D., Ph.D.,
of *Recovery Options: The Complete Guide*

"The material in *Mindful Recovery* offers mindfulness meditation as a powerful antidote to addiction as a 'disease' of the mind. Thomas and Beverly Bien have combined their professional experience as both therapists and practitioners of meditation in providing readers with a series of 'Doorways' into mindful recovery from addictive behaviors. . . .This is truly a book that opens many doors to greater awakening and self-awareness. The noted analyst Carl Jung once described many alcoholics as 'frustrated mystics' who were distracted in their quest by the 'spirits' in the bottle instead of pursuing the true pathway of spiritual awakening. Readers who identify with the frustrated-mystic group will find the path to spiritual liberation in the Doorways of this excellent book."

—from the foreword by G. Alan Marlatt, Ph.D.,
Professor of Psychology, Director, Addictive Behaviors
Research Center, University of Washington

Mindful Recovery

A Spiritual Path to

Healing from Addiction

Thomas Bien, Ph.D.
Beverly Bien, M.Ed.

John Wiley & Sons, Inc.

Published by John Wiley & Sons, Inc., New York
Published simultaneously in Canada

The author and publisher gratefully acknowledge the following sources for their permission to include copyrighted material: On page 10 from *The Way of Life According to Lao Tzu*, edited by Witter Bynner, copyright © 1944 by Witter Bynner. Copyright renewed © 1972 by Dorothy Chauvenet and Paul Horgan. Reprinted by permission of HarperCollins Publishers Inc. On page 114 from *The Enlightened Heart: An Anthology of Sacred Poetry*, by Wu-men, edited by Stephen Mitchell, copyright © 1989 by Stephen Mitchell. Reprinted by permission of Harper-Collins Publishers Inc. On pages 129–130 from *New Seeds of Contemplation* by Thomas Merton, copyright © 1961 by The Abbey of Gethsemani, Inc. Reprinted by permission of New Directions Publishing Corp. On page 215 from *Leaves of Grass* by Walt Whitman, edited with an introduction and notes by Jerome Loving (World's Classics, 1990). Used by permission of Oxford University Press.

This publication is designed to provide accurate and authoritative information in regard to the subject matter covered. It is sold with the understanding that the publisher is not engaged in rendering professional services. If professional advice or other expert assistance is required, the services of a competent professional person should be sought.

Library of Congress Cataloging-in-Publication Data

Bien, Thomas.
Mindful recovery: a spiritual path to healing from addiction / Thomas Bien, Beverly Bien.
p. cm.
Includes bibliographical references and index.
ISBN 0-471-44261-5
1. Substance abuse—Treatment. 2. Substance abuse—Religious aspects. 3. Meditation.
I. Bien, Beverly. II. Title.

RC564 .B54 2002
616.86'06—dc21   2001046863

Printed in the United States of America

10 9 8 7 6

To
Joshua Bien
and
Stacy Roalsen

The sage . . . accomplishes very much indeed because it is the *Tao* that acts in him and through him. He does not act of and by himself, still less for himself alone. His action is not a violent manipulation of exterior reality, an "attack" on the outside world, bending it to his conquering will: on the contrary, he respects external reality by yielding to it, and his yielding is at once an act of worship, a recognition of sacredness, and a perfect accomplishment of what is demanded by the precise situation.

—Thomas Merton, *Mystics and Zen Masters* (1967)

Contents

‿○‿

Foreword

❧

I once saw a cartoon that depicted two meditators seated next to each other, one a wizened old monk, the other a young novice with a perplexed expression on his face. The monk tells his young student, "Nothing happens next. This is it!"

For people who suffer from addictive behaviors, the present moment is never enough because the mind is focused on what happens next—the next "fix" is more important than accepting that "This is it" in the here and now of the present moment. As stated clearly throughout this fine book, *Mindful Recovery*, the practice of mindfulness or the development of what the authors describe as a "quality of calm awareness" is an excellent antidote for the addicted state of mind. It is as if the addicted individuals cannot accept the impermanence and change associated with moment-to-moment experience of life without "fixing" themselves by taking a substance or engaging in another addictive behavior in a vain attempt to create a permanent "high" that would provide an avoidance or escape from the painful "lows" of living.

In my own clinical practice with clients with addictive behavior problems, I have found meditation to be a powerful tool in relapse prevention. One client, a woman who came for therapy for co-occurring alcohol dependence and depression, decided to extend her practice by attending a ten-day meditation retreat. After the retreat was over, she told me that she had learned to accept and tolerate the endless pattern of urges and cravings that used to drive her to drink. In meditation, she came to observe the rise and fall of urges, as if they were waves on the sea, without being "wiped out" by them. She had learned the technique of "urge surfing," one of the practices described in this book. As she explained, she no longer felt "dictated to" by her urges to drink when she experienced painful emotions. She reminded me that the

Latin root for the term *addiction* is the same as for the word *dictator*. Instead of giving into the urge, as her mental dictator used to command, she was able to accept it as "just another thought" rising and falling like a wave passing through her mind. Meditation helped her think "outside of the box" of addicted thinking.

As a researcher, I have conducted several studies on the effects of meditation on addictive behaviors. In one study, we recruited heavy social drinkers who were willing to volunteer for a program that would teach them new ways to relax and manage stress. Participants were randomly assigned to one of three six-week training programs: meditation, deep muscle relaxation, or a control group who engaged in quiet reading for the same time periods as the meditation and muscle-relaxation groups (two twenty-minute periods a day). All participants were asked to keep track of their daily alcohol consumption during the six-week training program and for another six-week follow-up period during which they were free to continue practicing on their own if they so desired. We found that the drinkers in the meditation group decreased their alcohol consumption by fifty percent on the average, significantly more than participants in the other two groups. Not only did their drinking decrease; those in the meditation group opted to continue their daily practice significantly longer than other subjects during the follow-up period. Meditation appeared to work as a "positive addiction" that provided a relaxing alternative to daily drinking.

In our current research, we are evaluating the effect of a longer meditation course for individuals who have serious addiction problems and who have often failed in more traditional alcohol and substance-abuse treatment programs. Participants are volunteer inmates at a minimum-security prison located in Seattle, most of whom have a long history of drinking and drug problems, often combined with prostitution and burglary. The prison administration, working in conjunction with a local meditation center, recently introduced a ten-day meditation course for inmates who wished to learn about and practice Vipassana or insight-oriented meditation (based on a course first introduced in Indian prisons by S. N. Goenka, who serves as the primary teacher of this approach). The popularity of this course has been growing since it was first introduced in 1997, and more inmates are volunteering to participate. The goal of our study is to evaluate the impact of this intensive meditation course on alcohol and drug use (relapse rates) and re-arrest rates (recidivism) following release from the correctional facility. Inmates who complete the meditation course will be compared with a control group who did not volunteer for the course. Preliminary results indicate that participation in the mediation course is associated with a lowered recidivism rate, and that many participants reported new insights into the source of their drug/alcohol cravings and how to accept urges and temptations with greater equanimity and balance.

Several years ago, I attended a ten-day meditation retreat in northern California taught by S. N. Goenka, the same teacher who directs the prison meditation course described above. At the end of the course, I had the opportunity to ask him what he thought about how most Westerners defined addiction, such as alcoholism, as a physical (genetic or biological) disease. "Disease, yes," Goenka replied. "Addiction is a disease of the mind."

The material in *Mindful Recovery* offers mindfulness meditation as a powerful antidote to addiction as a "disease" of the mind. Thomas and Beverly Bien have combined their professional experience as both therapists and practitioners of meditation in providing readers with a series of "Doorways" into mindful recovery from addictive behaviors.

Each of the ten Doorway chapters opens up a new topic area in which to practice mindful living, ranging from discovering the magic of ordinary life experiences (Doorway One) to transforming negative emotional states (Doorway Nine). By combining personal case histories with active "homework assignments" and instructions for meditation practice, the authors describe a rich variety of options for enhancing awareness, developing greater self-acceptance and compassion for others, and awakening experience of one's own spiritual path.

I like how the authors describe these topics as a series of Doorways. As such, these ten Doorways offer a clear alternative to the traditional Twelve Steps of recovery as promoted by Alcoholics Anonymous and other Twelve-Step support groups. In the Buddhist model, the pathway out of the experience of suffering (including addiction) is described in the Four Noble Truths (described in Doorway One) as the Eightfold Path. Many of the branches of this Eightfold Path, including Right Mindfulness, are discovered and explored in the various Doorway chapters. In the Twelve-Step approach, members are told to take life "one day at a time." In the Buddhist model, this helpful adage is taken even further to experiencing life on a "moment-to-moment" level in the here and now (Doorway Ten).

This is truly a book that opens many doors to greater awakening and self-awareness. The noted analyst Carl Jung once described many alcoholics as "frustrated mystics" who were distracted in their quest by the "spirits" in the bottle instead of pursuing the true pathway of spiritual awakening. Readers who identify with the frustrated-mystic group will find the path to spiritual liberation in the Doorways of this excellent book.

G. Alan Marlatt, Ph.D.
Professor of Psychology
Director, Addictive Behaviors Research Center
University of Washington

Acknowledgments

❦

Buddhists are not alone in teaching that we are all deeply interconnected; so it is an obvious truth that a book is never truly the product of one person or even, as in this case, a pair of persons.

We gratefully acknowledge the support and comments of friends who suffered through early drafts, especially Russ Walsh, Ph.D., Joe Boroughs, Ph.D., Charles Elliott, Ph.D., and Pearl Gross, M.L.S. For unfailing encouragement and enthusiasm, Adam Balestrieri, M.A. For a productive brainstorming session over dinner we thank Tim Stryker, M.D., and Mikhal Stryker, M.A. For support and guidance regarding the business of writing, thanks to Bob Weber, Ph.D.

We also appreciate the efforts of Jeff Rutherford, formerly with the Denise Marcil Literary Agency, who helped shape our academic ramblings into something more readable, and our agents, Denise Marcil and Meredith Bernstein, who represented us with energy and ability. Our editor Tom Miller at Wiley offered numerous helpful ideas and suggestions. Also at Wiley, we thank Kimberly Monroe and Jude Patterson for their careful help in manuscript preparation.

Deep thanks to Professor G. Alan Marlatt of the University of Washington, profound scholar, researcher, and practicing Buddhist, for his contribution of the foreword to this text.

I (Tom) also thank my former teacher, renowned scholar-researcher Professor William Miller of the University of New Mexico, for all I learned from him about the scientific study of addictive behavior. Any errors in scholarship contained herein are, of course, mine.

We entreat the blessing of all high beings and bodhisattvas, that this work may ease the suffering of many.

PART ONE

❧

Mindful Recovery

Introduction

GETTING TO HERE AND NOW

The book you hold in your hands is the result of many years of reflection and study, experience and practice. Every page bears the mark of personal and professional struggle, as well as the peace that has since followed. This book brings together our lifelong interest in spirituality and spiritual practice with our professional interest in addiction.

I (Tom) have been studying the great spiritual traditions of the world for some time. It was over thirty years ago that I began practicing meditation and reading about Vedanta (the philosophy of the Vedas, the scriptures of Hinduism), the Upanishads, the Bhagavad Gita, the yoga aphorisms of Patanjali, and much more. These led to an increased openness also to Western spirituality, and then to a degree in theology. And while people often argue that their own brand of spirituality is the best if not the only true one, it seemed to me that those who practiced any form of spirituality in depth were pointing to the same underlying reality.

In pursuing a doctorate in psychology, I developed a focus in the field of addictive behavior. This was a great area for learning about how human beings change or fail to change, and about that basic human dilemma that, even when we know we are doing something harmful and destructive, we cannot always manage to put that insight into practice. As my spirituality turned toward Buddhism in general and mindfulness in particular, and as my professional work led me

3

deeper into the practice of psychotherapy, the sense began to emerge that these interests had a lot to say to each other. Therapy itself, or so it seems to me, is a form of mindfulness practice. Over the years I have come increasingly to connect my work with clients and mindfulness practice—first of all for myself, deepening my own level of presence in sessions, but also in talking to clients about conscious breathing, meditation, and becoming more deeply and calmly present in their lives.

Beverly's path also led her into spiritual practice and therapy with an addictions focus: her initial interest in addictions arose through personal experience. In an alcoholic first marriage, she saw firsthand the impact that alcohol can have on one's life. After coming through her own addiction to nicotine, her interest in addictions intensified and she created and taught a behaviorally based smoking-cessation program. With a master's degree in counseling psychology, she has worked for over twelve years in human services and education with diverse populations, including adults with severe mental illness, homeless substance-abusing adults, and incarcerated mentally ill and substance-abusing adults.

Dealing with the problems of the severely mentally ill is difficult and draining, and Beverly soon experienced a need for a deeper spiritual awareness and practice. She began making retreats to re-center herself and incorporated meditation and yoga into her life. When she and I entered each other's lives some seven years ago, we discovered that we had these interests in common. We supported each other in deepening our own practice of mindfulness and, once we had gained some stability and insight, in sharing the fruit of this with others through our Mindful Living workshops. Over time, the idea for this book took clear shape.

Awareness, the Common Denominator

At heart, we saw that the common thread in all these interests was a certain quality of calm awareness—what the Buddhists call mindfulness. We experienced both our clients and ourselves growing in ability to face life and deal with it deeply and effectively. Mindfulness seemed the natural antidote for many problems involved in addiction, which is at its core a way of *avoiding* life rather than being aware of it. For many addicted people, addictive behavior is a way to turn problems off for a while. Unfortunately, of course, doing this increases both the number and the complexity of their problems. And while many have found spirituality and meaning to be key in leaving addiction behind, it seemed natural to us to consider that a spirituality based specifically on mindfulness—which is the opposite of avoiding—would offer something uniquely helpful to those who struggled with addiction.

Over time the insight that a spirituality of mindfulness could be especially helpful to addicted people gathered weight and substance. And while our approach is psychologically informed, we did not want to offer another form of therapy per se, but a *spiritual approach to life* that would help addicted people face their lives and rebuild them with greater clarity and calm, greater peace and insight. We offer a spiritual path for those who, already having begun the process of change, now seek a spiritual foundation to continue to build upon.

A Spiritual Path

When we describe our approach as a spiritual path, we do not intend a narrow or restrictive understanding of spirituality, but rather a broad and inclusive one. The word itself is based on the word *spirit*, as in Holy Spirit or Spirit of God. We intend a connection with these meanings. The words for spirit in both Hebrew (*ruach*) and Greek (*pneuma*), the primary languages of the Bible, have additional meanings of breath or wind. The word *spiritus* in Latin has these same meanings. In the Genesis story of Creation, God breathes into the lifeless human form of Adam, and Adam, filled now with God's breath/spirit, becomes a living being. This implies that the *élan vital*, or vital force in us, is directly related to the Divine. It also hints at the importance of the breath in spiritual practice.

We recognize that for some, however, all of the implications of "spiritual" as something connected with God or a Divine Being present a barrier. It is not necessary to subscribe to notions of a personal deity to benefit from this book. If these connections are not helpful to you, consider the following suggestions: (1) By the word *spiritual*, we mean also a sense of the poetry of life, *your* sense of life's beauty and movement and meaning. You may have a spiritual moment when you see your newborn child open his eyes for the first time, or when you watch a sunset or see a woman comb her hair, or when you touch the ancient stones of some ruin. You can have such moments of epiphany riding a horse, or surfing, or planting flowers if that is your passion, or in speaking simply and directly from the heart to another person. (2) By the word *spiritual*, we mean something close also to the word *existential*. In the practice of the Five Remembrances, Buddhists remind themselves that their deeds are their only true possession. That is not only a page straight out of Sartre, but a much older page, preceding existentialism by some twenty-five hundred years. It includes an awareness that life is limited and therefore precious, that we must fill each moment with a meaning of our choosing. It is a sense also that the choices we make are important and that we must make them with awareness, since each turn in the road limits future alternatives.

Why Buddhism?

It is a symptom of our own cultural limitations that most of us inevitably think of one religion as against another, one spiritual path in opposition to all other varieties. But what Beverly and I have in mind is not to make people Buddhists in the sense of no longer being a Christian or a Jew or even an agnostic for that matter. Buddhism is not a religion or a philosophy in our Western sense of the word, but a *path of liberation*. Siddhartha Gautama, who became the Buddha, was not interested in starting a religion to compete with others in the religious marketplace. He was not interested in philosophical or metaphysical speculation. In fact, when he was asked about such things—things like the origin of the universe, for instance—he usually remained silent. So when you hear about Buddhist teachings, it is important to keep them in this context. Though it may sound sometimes like a religion or a philosophy, this is not the essence of Buddhism at all. It is about practice. It is about how to live in a way that ends suffering and brings peace and freedom.

Gautama had been through the whole religious and spiritual gamut available in his time and place, in India some five hundred years B.C. He pursued them all to their ultimate depth and conclusion, and found them all wanting. When he reached that state called nirvana or enlightenment, he had touched something beyond all these teachings, beliefs, and practices. It was not immediately apparent to him that he should try to teach anyone anything, or even try to talk about his experience at all. At first he was content to go on as a silent sage. But before long he realized that this was not enough. As he observed the suffering of nonenlightened beings, he knew he had to do what he could to alleviate their suffering. He knew he had to try to help. So he spoke up and started teaching. And at the end of his life, after teaching for many years, he maintained that everything he had ever said was only about *suffering and the cessation of suffering*. This was his sole interest as a teacher.

The heart of the Buddha's teaching is the Four Noble Truths—which are completely about suffering and how to end it:

1. The First Noble Truth is that *suffering is*. The Buddha does not say that all of life is suffering, but calls attention to the very thing we want to ignore. The word *dukkha*, translated as "suffering," may better be translated as the unsatisfactoriness of things, or the frustration of living, because it is not just about catastrophic experiences like terminal illness and death, but includes the difficulty of finding a parking place and figuring out what kind of a job to pursue.
2. The Second Noble Truth concerns the cause of suffering. In essence, this means that, while life is continually changing and impermanent, we refuse to make peace with this fact, but try to act as though we can hold on.
3. The Third Noble Truth teaches that there is a way out of this frustrating situation, a way to let go.
4. The Fourth Noble Truth describes what the kind of life that releases us from suffering looks like.

The kind of life leading out of suffering, as described in the Fourth Noble Truth, is the Eightfold Path: Right View, Right Thinking, Right Speech, Right Action, Right Livelihood, Right Mindfulness, Right Diligence, and Right Concentration. Each of the eight aspects is proceeded by the same Pali word (*samyak*), usually translated as "right." But it would be a mistake to understand this primarily as right in the moral sense, as Westerners raised on the Ten Commandments are liable to do. The Buddha's focus was practical, not moral or speculative. The word *right* is best taken in the sense of whole or complete or effective. In other words, this is simply how to live so as to escape from the net of suffering. These eight areas work together in such a way that to practice any one of them deeply involves the practice of all the others as well. It is impossible, for example, to have right insight without its being connected with what you do at work, how you talk to others, and so forth. That is, Right View leads in the direction of Right Livelihood and Right Speech. Given this interconnectedness, it is possible to simplify, and focus on mindfulness alone, since this inevitably includes the rest as well.

The attitude in Buddhism is, if you want to find a way out of suffering, try these practices and see for yourself. Don't accept them on faith or any such thing—except the kind of provisional faith you need to give something a real try in the first place. But check it out and see. It is a highly practical attitude.

We think it is quite possible for our readers to remain committed Christians, Jews, Muslims, or agnostics and use the practices presented in this book. As your understanding of the path of mindfulness deepens, you will resonate more deeply with mindfulness aspects of your own tradition—for example, when Jesus teaches not to worry about tomorrow, but to let the day's own trouble be sufficient for the day.

Addiction

Most of us generally use the word *addiction* in its narrow, original sense of a problematic and destructive pattern of use of a substance or chemical in which the body becomes adjusted to the presence of that substance. When the person who is addicted in this sense, then abruptly stops use of that substance, he experiences an abnormal state called withdrawal.

It has become common, however, to use the word *addiction* in an extended and metaphorical sense whenever there is a compulsive quality about a behavior pattern. Nowadays people speak about addiction to work, sex, or food. This metaphorical use does bring out a certain truth about these kinds of problematic behaviors, so Beverly and I feel no need in what is at heart a spiritual book to insist on a narrow definition. Many people whose problems involve this more extended kind of addiction will find help here as well.

A Word about Our Stories

While the people in our stories are true to life in the sense of being based on our experiences in therapy and elsewhere, they are generally composites, based on several people rather than one single individual. In those cases where they are based primarily on a single individual, identifying characteristics have been altered to preserve anonymity. Also, throughout the book, rather than use the pronoun *he* to represent a person of either gender, we alternate between the pronouns *he* and *she*.

The Process of Change

People through finding something beautiful
Think something else unbeautiful,
Through finding one man fit
Judge another unfit.
—Lao-tzu, *The Way of Life*, 6th century B.C.

A Life Almost Lost: Melissa's Story

"I was never going to touch a drop. I saw what alcohol did to my parents' lives. I can still hear the screaming and shouting that went on almost daily. My sister and I used to hug each other to sleep, night after night. I always knew that if I ever started drinking, I would never stop."

Melissa's prophecy eventually came true. Urged on by friends at a college party, she finally succumbed. "My first drink actually didn't taste that good, but I still went for the second." Despite the taste, she immediately knew her relationship to alcohol would be a long one. Soon Melissa began drinking regularly at dormitory parties and lived up to her expectations of herself. "The days blended into each other. There were more parties. At first they were a lot of fun. But I slacked off on studying. I began to skip class because I was so hung over. And of course my grades fell. I was flunking everything and feeling anxious all the time. The anxiety became a problem in itself—another reason to say the hell with it, and just drink some more. I dropped out of school in the middle of my sophomore year and just took a boring clerical job in an insurance office."

Her dreams coming to a grinding halt, Melissa suffered from a lack of meaning and purpose in life. At one time her spiritual interests and passion for helping others might have led her to a career in mental health—the life dream of her adolescence. But instead, her spiritual yearning became a hazy, alcoholic path, searching for answers in an altered state of consciousness.

On a number of occasions, Melissa came close to death while driving in an intoxicated state. The real tragedy for her, however, was not to be so dramatic as a fatal car crash. Her tragedy was more about the deadly dullness that attends unfulfilled dreams. Alcohol rerouted her onto a path of unsatisfying career choices, destructive relationships, and physical deterioration. Her life was stuck. She took a series of clerical positions well beneath her abilities and never seemed able to get back on track. As she put it, "Every day has been a struggle to get through. Nothing makes sense. I still consider going into mental health, but I get completely overwhelmed just thinking about it. So, what do I do? I pour myself another drink."

When Melissa came in for her first therapy session, she had stopped drinking for about three weeks. We talked about basic principles: that addiction is often a matter of running away from something that hurts, and that this in turn creates many other problems. She agreed with this in an abstract kind of way. But it was clear that she did not connect these ideas to her own experience at first. In the first few meetings, it was hard for Melissa to reveal much of herself. Whenever she seemed to get close to her pain, she immediately ran from it or tried to neutralize it. For example, she said: "I'm not really happy with the kind of work I'm doing. There's a feeling that I could be doing more, somehow." But immediately she added: "But I suppose everyone feels that way." Then she went on to other, safer topics.

Gradually, she became more capable of befriending her pain. We discussed meditation as a way of learning to be with thoughts and feelings without getting caught up in them. Progress in therapy accelerated when she started meditating. She began to notice how she ran away from her pain the moment it surfaced, and started to see that painful thoughts and feelings often triggered a relapse urge.

As another tool, Melissa started journaling. Through writing in her journal, she began to see life patterns. She realized that she had always been a bit of a Goody Two-shoes. She was the kind of child who loved to be chosen class monitor when the teacher left the room, and who was mortified the time she got her first C on her report card. She started to see that drinking gave her an excuse to relax and be a little wild, a little rebellious. Over time, she came to own her need to let go and have fun, but to do this in less destructive ways.

Toward the end of therapy, she started to talk about her all but forgotten dream to be a counselor. Though she could not afford to go back to school just then, she found a job at a psychiatric hospital as a mental health worker. This represented a cut in pay from her clerical work at first, but she found it more satisfying. There were problems with the institution she worked for, and the state was always threatening further cutbacks in the budget. But somehow she carried these problems differently than problems in her other jobs. They were problems on her own path. In our last meeting, she had begun to consider how she could get additional training and credentials.

Heeding the Signal

Putting your life back together after wrestling loose from an addiction is a gradual process. Melissa is not alone in being able to slowly put the pieces back together. Nor is she alone in losing her way in life. If you are not on your path, there can be a gnawing pain and emptiness in you. What do you fill yourself with? How do you fill your time? How do you occupy your body and mind? Though you may want to run from the pain, pain is a signal that something is wrong, that something needs attention and healing. As a signal, it is valuable, though its lessons hurt.

One of the most important aspects of the art of living is how we deal with pain—especially emotional pain. Will we heed its lessons, or, in desperation, do anything to turn it off—even temporarily? Will we be present to the emptiness, or will we seek to fill it at all costs? Some people try to fill that pain and emptiness with consumerism, ambition, or an endless flow of romantic adventures. Some try to fill it with television, with work and busyness, with computers or video games, never allowing any space. And some try to fill it with drugs like alcohol, as Melissa did.

Are You Already Full?

While programs for addiction can be found nearly everywhere, it is clear these are not entirely meeting the vast need. This book is for those who are seeking a spiritual view of life to help understand their addiction, but are not entirely content with the spirituality currently offered in mainstream programs. Abstinence is a great first step in the recovery process. But when you eliminate something that was so much a part of your life, you need to be open to the spiritual dimension to help you through the resulting changes.

A Buddhist story illustrates the need for openness. A student approached a famous Zen master for instruction. The student tried to impress the master with his knowledge of Buddhism, and discoursed endlessly from his vast intellectual knowledge of the subject. The master poured tea into the student's cup, and continued to pour over his protests even after it started to overflow. It was impossible, the master said, to give Zen to someone who was already full, already certain of knowing the truth.

If you are open, if your cup is not already full, we will gently guide you toward a path of mindful recovery. Together we will explore the spiritual and emotional impact of leaving addiction behind.

Mindfulness

The connection between addiction and spirituality is ancient and venerable. To date, the spirituality of recovery has been influenced primarily by Western religious thinking. And though people seem increasingly interested in the spirituality of the East, little has been done to connect these traditions with the needs of people who struggle with addiction.

Our approach is based on the Buddhist teaching of mindfulness. Mindfulness is a quality of openness, of present-moment awareness and acceptance. Mindfulness is experiencing this moment, this very one, the only moment that exists. Mindful living is not about living in the future or dwelling in the past. It is also not about recriminations when you find yourself in the past or the future. Mindfulness is about getting back in touch with your spiritual essence, your true nature.

Mindfulness allows you to be open to your pain so you can learn its lessons and get your life back into harmony, into Tao. You do not have to become a Buddhist or desert your own religious heritage to practice mindfulness. In fact, you do not need to be religious at all in the usual sense. *Mindful Recovery* looks at addiction and explores a more harmonious path to recovery. Because addicted people get caught in unawareness, using drugs rather than face what hurts, mindfulness provides a gentle way to begin to face the pain.

Mindfulness helps in two ways. First, by being mindful, by being aware of the state of your body, emotions, and environment, you receive clear signals concerning what is out of balance and what hurts. When you learn to respect these signals and welcome them rather than push them away, you no longer need to turn the signal off by indulging. You therefore become less likely to continue the destructive, automatic behaviors involved in addiction.

Mindfulness also helps by putting you back in touch with the simple pleasure of being alive. As Rabbi Abraham Heschel said, "Just to be is a blessing. Just to live is holy." Each moment contains a potential fullness—a simple satisfaction in living—that refreshes the spirit. You need only be open to it. But this opening is difficult for the addicted person, for addiction is about blunting your perceptions, about closing off. And though it may be motivated by a desire to close off to things that hurt, it also closes you off to the refreshment of simple, present-moment experiences: the cool of the morning, a dog barking a greeting, the comfort of your favorite chair. By putting you back in touch with simple pleasures, mindfulness reduces the need to fill the void with drugs and other destructive things.

Flowers by the Road

Mindfulness of the world beyond ourselves and our thoughts, in its richness and color and drama, makes it unnecessary to enhance our lives artificially, filling our emptiness with drugs. Most of us reject this richer awareness, however, because it does not always conform to our idea of how things *should be* and what we *should* pay attention to. If in driving to work all you are aware of is the pressure to get there on time, you will not notice the other people around you, the sensations of brisk, invigorating cold on a winter morning or the ovenlike, soporific warmth in summer, or the glorious sunrise or mountains or ocean or green trees or expanse of desert. Of course you can't forget that you have to get to work! But if you can tune in to these other, nonutilitarian aspects as well, the experience of driving to work becomes full *in itself*—a means to an end, surely, but no longer *just* a means to an end.

Meditation teacher and author Sharon Salzberg tells the story of one of her teachers who was asked why he meditated. The students waited expectantly for his words, anticipating some deep, esoteric wisdom. He replied that he meditated not to miss the little purple flowers by the side of the road. Mindfulness is about the little things.

To illustrate this kind of awareness, Buddhist teacher Thich Nhat Hanh gives the example of doing the dishes just to do the dishes. If you are doing the dishes in order to be able to go on to something you think will be more satisfying than doing the dishes, not only will you not enjoy doing the dishes, but you will not enjoy whatever it is you go on to do next. If you are doing the dishes just to get to your dessert, then you won't enjoy dessert either. For while you are eating your dessert, your mind will again be racing ahead to the next thing—to the video you've rented, the phone call you need to make, or the novel you want to finish. In this way, you fail to live the actual moments of your life because you are instead always trying to get to some other, better moment. You never live, but are always planning to live.

The Need for Clear Experiencing

As food nourishes the body, so experience nourishes the spirit. We all need the richness of direct, clear experience. It keeps the soul healthy and well nourished. When we do not get this food because our experience is blocked by anxieties, fears, worries, and plans, the soul becomes anemic. Psychologists have conducted many studies with what is known as a sensory deprivation tank. This is a small, dark, sound-insulated compartment partly filled with salt water warmed to body temperature like the womb. The subject enters the compartment and stays in for long periods to explore the effect this has on human functioning and perception. Subjects who remain in these tanks for long periods often begin to hallucinate. The brain, being starved for stimulation, creates its own.

When we are not mindful, when we are not getting the experiential food we need, we get a little crazy. We become psychologically starved. We are plagued by all manner of imaginings and fears having little to do with reality. Worse still, we can run around trying to seek intense stimulation to feed our starving minds. Some people try to do this through drugs and alcohol, rather than by tuning in to the wealth of experience already at hand. But this is a kind of junk food to the mind, filling but not nourishing. They become like people starving in a grocery store filled with food.

Using Western Tools

Eastern spiritual traditions—especially those which emphasize a here-and-now awareness or mindfulness—offer a helpful perspective on addiction. The automatic, compulsive quality of addiction is incompatible with the open spaciousness of a merciful, gentle mindfulness. Where mindfulness is, addiction is not. Where addiction is, mindfulness is not. Cultivation of one leaves less room for the other.

While our approach is rooted in Eastern traditions of mindfulness in its overall spirit and intention, this does not mean that all of the actual techniques have to come from far away. The West has its own approaches to mindfulness. Journaling, narrative psychology, insight-oriented psychotherapy, relationship work, and dream analysis are all tools that have been developed in the West. All of these approaches also create an increased awareness and openness. These techniques have the added advantage of being rooted in our own culture, and are therefore in some ways easier for Westerners to understand. Unlike books about mindfulness rooted solely in traditional Eastern techniques, we present a blend of Eastern and Western wisdom.

Though many models of recovery perpetuate a disease-based focus, we promote a health-based model. That is, we emphasize building on health and strength rather than disease or pathology. Our approach is about facing what hurts and finding answers. We emphasize staying in contact with the positive aspects of life, and living a full, satisfying, meaningful life rather than focusing on sickness or powerlessness. Only by touching the parts of life that are healthy and positive will any of us find the strength to confront our problems.

Black-and-White Thinking

One example of how a disease focus can actually contribute to the problem is the abstinence violation effect, or AVE. The AVE is a type of black-and-white thinking. It is similar to the AA slogan, "one drink, one drunk." The AVE says that recovering individuals view themselves as either completely sober on the one hand, or completely out of control on the other, with no in between. This view creates a lot of problems. For the alcoholic who believes that one drink inevitably and always results in one drunk, and who then has a slip, there will be a greater inclination to engage in self-defeating thinking such as, "I'm a no-good, hopeless drunk. The disease has got me, and I can't do anything about it. As they say, I'm powerless." Thinking this way, of course, increases the probability that she will continue to drink destructively. In other words, it becomes a self-fulfilling prophecy. And while it is good to be cautious and avoid slips when possible, this radically polarized view helps ensure that a slip becomes a fall, that one drink will inevitably lead to full-blown relapse.

Mindfulness helps you to see the signals leading to a slip, and also helps you to recognize one drink as just that: one drink. Practicing mindfulness, you are more likely to avoid falling off the wagon in the first place, and you are also less likely to exaggerate the importance of a slip, less likely to see it as ultimate defeat or failure.

How We Change

There are distinctive needs in overcoming addictive or other forms of habitual behavior. The first need is to mobilize resources to stop the behavior: But beyond this there is a need to find a way of maintaining this new state. Recall Mark Twain's comment about quitting smoking.

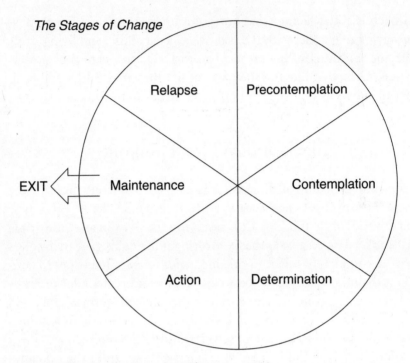

The Stages of Change

Adapted from Prochaska and DiClemente, 1982.

"To cease smoking is the easiest thing," he said. "I've done it a thousand times." To be successful, you need to do more than just quit. You need to stay that way!

To put this in a larger context, there are distinct stages of change in recovery. In each stage, distinctive needs must be met to progress to the next stage. The stages psychologists James Prochaska and Carlo DiClemente have shown in their research are precontemplation (being unaware of a problem), contemplation (questioning if there might be a problem), determination (deciding to change), action (quitting), maintenance (staying quit), and relapse. Often an individual can go through this cycle several times, relapsing and quitting again, before finally exiting the process and resting steadily in the new, sober way of being.

In order for an addicted person—an alcoholic, for example—to move from the precontemplation stage, where he is totally unaware that there is a problem, to the contemplation stage, something must happen that poses the possibility that a problem exists. He may notice friends with a similar problem, see a relative falling seriously ill because of alcohol, or may simply notice his anxiety mount when he runs low on alcohol.

In the contemplation stage, the person is not *convinced* she has a problem, but is only aware there *might* be. Internally, you can think of this person as seesawing between thinking there is a problem and feeling there is no problem. The inner dialogue of someone with a drinking problem might sound like this: "I really have to change my drinking. I'm tired of waking up feeling horrible, having to face another day with a headache and a queasy stomach. But on the other hand, I know lots of people who drink as much as I do—or even more! If I'm so bad, what about Charlie? What about Sue? Maybe it's okay. I'm just having fun, after all. Just letting off some steam. Still, though, I hated the way my son looked at me the other night when I was drunk . . . "—and so forth. To move on from this stage requires some convincing event or information, something that overcomes this ambivalence and seesawing.

One client moved on from the contemplation phase when he found himself at the corner store with enough money for a pack of cigarettes, but not enough for both the cigarettes and some milk for his toddler. He bought the cigarettes instead of the milk. This astonishing act startled him into awareness that he clearly had a problem.

Once you are convinced you have a problem, a window for change opens called the determination stage. To take advantage of this opening requires a plan for change that feels realistic. Your thoughts might be, "I will quit smoking on the first of the month. I will throw all my remaining cigarettes away in ritual fashion. I will write down all the reasons I want to quit, and whenever I am tempted, I will take out that list of reasons and read it to remind myself." If no realistic plan emerges, the window closes, and you are likely to find yourself back in precontemplation, telling yourself it's really not that serious.

If you acknowledge the need to change, and can envision a way to carry it out, you enter the action stage. This is a matter of putting the plan into practice, of doing whatever you need to do to quit. In maintenance, however, the needs are quite different. To be successful in this stage, and to ultimately exit the cycle altogether, you need different skills—ones that help you stay quit rather than help you quit, per se.

To negotiate the maintenance stage, you need perseverance. You need the capacity to adjust your skills to changing situations, including ones you had not anticipated.

Stan, for example, had managed to stop drinking for six months. He did this by avoiding high-risk situations, places where he knew alcohol would be readily available and offered to him. However, now he faces the prospect of his brother's wedding, and he knows there will be plenty of alcohol at the reception. Because he wants to support his brother by attending the wedding, his strategy of avoiding risky situations will be inadequate for this. To deal with this type of problem, he needs a way to be around alcohol and still not drink. If he does not find a way to do so, he will enter relapse and go back to the beginning of the cycle, being unaware of having a problem (precontemplation).

It is of great help in staying quit or successfully negotiating the maintenance stage to have a larger focus for your life. This larger focus can be anything from spiritual commitment or service, to things that are much more ordinary. Unsuccessful negotiation of the maintenance stage leads to relapse, and then back to precontemplation.

Most people go through this cycle several times before exiting entirely into sober, healthy living. Very likely, you have known someone who has done this, or have done it yourself. However, this obvious-sounding observation is actually very important. For *recovery is a process*. It is a process of navigating between complacency on the one hand, and self-recrimination and despair on the other. Many know the danger of complacency. They know that relapse is a serious business, in some cases even life-threatening. It is obviously something to avoid if possible. At the same time, though, most people do go through these stages several times before establishing permanent change. For this reason, it is equally important to be able to view a slip, once it occurs, as a temporary setback rather than ultimate failure. Expecting yourself to get it right the first time out can be as unrealistic as expecting to hit a home run your first time at bat: it happens, but it is one for the record books, not the usual way of things. So when a slip does occur, it is important to maintain a compassionate attitude toward yourself, seeing yourself as in a learning process rather than doomed to failure. You are human, and this is the way human beings learn. By bringing mindfulness to the slip and what triggered it, you can form a plan to deal with that kind of situation in future.

This book primarily addresses the needs of people in the maintenance phase. That is, *it will show you how to build a satisfying and meaningful way of life without addiction once you have quit.* After contemplating quitting an addiction, after the decision has been made and implemented, there remains this tedious business of living without the alcohol or other drug. This part deserves special attention. For if you can build a happy, fulfilling, meaningful life, relapse will be much less of an issue.

A Larger Purpose

Mindfulness provides a larger purpose. When you have a larger purpose, a broader context in which to see a problem, things fall into place more gently, more easily. If you are awake and relaxed and aware and enjoying your life, there will be both less need and less desire for drugs, or anything else that you lean on too heavily.

Goals other than mindfulness can provide that larger context which gives us greater resilience and greater enjoyment of the present. For example, people who become interested in health and fitness often find they change other habits such as eating and drinking in order to support the larger goal of health. The Higher Power of the Twelve Steps has worked this way for some. Existential psychologist Viktor Frankl survived the horror of a Nazi concentration camp by having the larger purpose of observing and recording his experiences. He was fond of quoting Nietzsche's dictum, "He who has a *why* to live can bear with almost any *how*."

Awareness or mindfulness itself can be just such an overarching goal. Whether the day ahead presents a busy round of work, or a peaceful day at the beach, the mindfulness practitioner approaches it the same way, with an intention to be aware, to experience fully and deeply. We are the eyes and ears of the universe; we must not cloud our vision or muffle our hearing.

The Tao of Golf: Martin's Story

A larger purpose need not be lofty, spiritual, or overtly religious. For Martin, golf became a means of practicing mindfulness. He had already quit several times. He would quit his cocaine use successfully for a few weeks, but then start again. During one of his periods of abstinence, a friend invited him to play golf. His friend was a patient teacher, and Martin came to love the game. He loved everything about it: being outside with friends, strolling over the carefully manicured greens, the grace of a swing that flowed naturally and easily as he improved. But one time he had to play while recovering from a coke binge the previous evening. He played terribly and felt worse. That was it. Though cocaine had cost him two jobs and his marriage to Katherine, it was his newly acquired sport that motivated him to become drug free. For him, what was important was that nothing interfere with his golf game. As his passion for golf increased, his passion for cocaine decreased.

Martin's story also points out that while quitting is an essential step, it is not enough. One needs a new focus. While other things can provide it, in our view, the best focus you can have is on living more deeply, more spiritually. In this book, we offer mindfulness as just such a focus—indeed, as a way of life. We offer specific strategies to help you *create a lifestyle that, by its nature, discourages addiction.* To set your feet on a path that is intrinsically healing, we present the ten Doorways to mindfulness.

The Ten Doorways to Mindfulness

Doorway One: *Return to the present moment.* You can get overwhelmed by memories of the past, worries about the future, and other distractions. When that happens, you may be in danger of relapse. By bringing a gentle, compassionate awareness to your surroundings, your thoughts, and your feelings, you will discover that your need to engage in addictive behavior diminishes.

Doorway Two: *Consider your life as a story you are still writing.* Many people hold on to life scripts connected to their addiction, which perpetuate negative life stories as well as continued attraction to drugs and alcohol. You don't have to get stuck there. You can write a new story.

Doorway Three: *Use journaling to deepen awareness of your life story and open the door to spiritual awakening.* Regular journaling brings the power of mindfulness to bear on repetitive problems and aids in contacting your inner wisdom.

Doorway Four: *Practice meditation to become more accepting of yourself and your life.* When you become more accepting of what hurts as well as more aware of life's many positive aspects, you establish a firm spiritual foundation for recovery.

Doorway Five: *Find ways to connect with the natural world.* Addicted people are often alienated from the natural world. A return to nature is incompatible with addiction. Conscious, mindful choices about your recreational time prevent you from squandering it on passive pursuits that do not employ your higher human qualities, such as intellectual, artistic, and spiritual activities.

Doorway Six: *Cultivate healthy relationships to discourage addiction.* Many people become addicted in part because of painful and unsatisfying relationships. In turn, addiction can destroy even the best relationship. As you become more mindful of relationship patterns, you can begin to change them, reducing the need to indulge your addiction.

Doorway Seven: *Explore dreams to expand your view of who you are beyond the limited point of view of your conscious, rational self.* Dreams offer clues about what is missing and what is out of balance. Often these are blind spots which we have difficulty seeing consciously.

Doorway Eight: *Practice mindfulness at work.* A mindful life involves mindfulness in all areas of life. Practicing mindfulness at work can help you stay calm and centered there as well.

Doorway Nine: *Learn to hold and embrace difficult emotions to ensure successful recovery.* There are well-established methods for dealing with difficult feelings. If you need extra help, therapy may be a useful aid.

Doorway Ten: *Practice, practice, practice.* An intellectual understanding of how to change your life is just the beginning. Direct experience brings the peace, health, and wholeness you seek.

Just One Way?

While it is not so everywhere else, in North America the predominant approach to the treatment of addiction remains Alcoholics Anonymous and its related Twelve-Step groups and programs. Individual stories attesting to the helpfulness of AA and Twelve Steps are numerous. Many people know someone who has been helped by a Twelve-Step program.

But is that all there is? The dominance of this one point of view is a two-edged sword—helpful to some, but also limiting the acceptance and development of alternative views with something to offer.

The problem with valuing one thing so much is that our attachment to it then makes it difficult to value anything else. The ancient sage Lao-tzu, credited with authorship of the Tao-Te Ching (pronounced Dow Deh Jing, sometimes translated as "The Way of Life") and the founder of Taoism, wrote the words at the beginning of this chapter some time around the sixth century B.C. Because you find one thing helpful, do you have to reject everything else? Because you find one thing helpful, does that exhaust all possibilities?

Lao-tzu's words teach us that because one thing is good or beautiful or helpful, this should not preclude other things from also being good or beautiful or helpful. A both-and approach is often more useful and more complete than an either-or approach.

Whether you have found other programs helpful or not, our hope is that this book can give you something different, something that may *also* be helpful to you. If you approach this book with an empty cup, with openness, you will find things of value, without having to give up what you already have. And if, on the other hand, you have not yet found what you need elsewhere, we hope this book gives you a useful perspective, and helps you find the courage and strength to change.

PART TWO

The Ten Doorways to Mindful Recovery

Doorway One

SEEING THE MAGIC
OF THE ORDINARY

The foundation of happiness is mindfulness. The basic
condition for being happy is our consciousness of being
happy. If we are not aware that we are happy, we are not
really happy. When we have a toothache, we know that not
having a toothache is a wonderful thing. But when we do not
have a toothache, we are still not happy.
—Thich Nhat Hanh, *Peace Is Every Step* (1991)

✧

*Return to the present moment. You can get overwhelmed by memo-
ries of the past, worries about the future, and other distractions.
When that happens, you may be in danger of relapse. By bringing a
gentle, compassionate awareness to your surroundings, your thoughts,
and your feelings, you will discover that your need to engage in
addictive behavior diminishes.*

✧

Taking Care of the Present: Tim's Story

"I just didn't see it slipping away," Tim said. He had thought life was going well. He had a secure job, a loving family, money invested for retirement, and the respect of his community. Though he drank heavily every night, and even more on weekends, and though this often resulted in a horrible argument with his wife, somehow he ignored this. Life was good—until one day his wife and adolescent daughter left him. And all of a sudden, as it seemed, Tim found himself in my office.

Of course, things had actually been getting worse for years. Tim's alcoholism had been stalking him silently and steadily for a long time. As blood vessels to the heart accumulate blockage slowly, bit by bit, and everything may seem fine until the moment the heart attack strikes, so the effects of Tim's drinking had been quietly piling up, slowly, steadily, perniciously. It seemed sudden to Tim only because he had been so unaware.

Tim had been living in forgetfulness, out of touch with the reality of his life. Now he would have to learn in therapy to take better care of his life, of each precious moment. If Tim cannot learn it now, his life will spiral out of control, drifting deeper and deeper into difficulty and suffering. Only if he learns to take care of the future by caring for the present will he emerge intact.

Where Are You?

Tim needs to learn to come into the present and be where he is. He comes into therapy like the Zen student who asks the master how he may achieve enlightenment. The master responds: "Where are you?" In other words, enlightenment is not some *thing* that you can grasp and claim like a trophy. Enlightenment is being where you are, being present. Right here. Right now. Tim has to start where he is.

To be mindful is to be gently aware. There is a richness in each moment that, when viewed with a quiet, compassionate attention, yields a fascinated contentment. Touching this reality, one understands the ancient author of the Upanishads who, describing it, was reduced to repeated exclamations: "Oh, Wonderful! Wonderful! Wonderful!"

There are different kinds of awareness. We can be aware, but be in protest. Like the two-year-old stamping her feet and screaming, "No!" we can be at war with the world. Or we can have a goal-oriented awareness, an awareness that narrows in scope to only those features of our world which serve to meet the goal. We can have an awareness that is cold, detached, analytical, like a technician looking at tumor cells under a microscope, forgetting that these cells were taken from a living person. Or we can think of the scolding teacher who told us, "Pay attention!" and confuse this with mindfulness.

None of this is mindfulness. Nor does mindfulness mean a shallow philosophy of living for the day, as if you had no past and no responsibility toward the future. Mindfulness heals the past and cares for the future in the only time in which it is possible to do this: the present moment.

Pain and Pleasure

Human beings are hardwired to avoid pain and seek pleasure. For the most part, this characteristic is helpful. It gives us a built-in tendency to seek things that are good for us and avoid dangers. However, this same tendency can also get us into trouble. Whereas a person who is already in shape will love exercise, find that it actually feels good, and therefore continue to seek it out, the average American couch potato dislikes all the heavy breathing and sweating and sore muscles. To get in shape and become someone who finds exercise pleasurable, you have to get used to these strange sensations, and allow your body and mind to adjust to a higher level of activity.

Drug addiction reveals how our tendency to seek pleasure and avoid pain can go awry. Addicted individuals seek the easy way out. They learn to turn off their pain by dulling it, rather than face it, learn its lessons, and do something to make things better. The difficulty is compounded by the intense but short pleasure that drugs provide.

Mindfulness is quite different. Mindfulness is detached in the sense that our focus is not narrowed solely by our desire to seek pleasure and avoid pain. It is a warm, caring awareness. It is compassion toward self and others. It is an awareness that finds delight in what is, and is not so completely occupied with what we think should be. It is an awareness that is soft and open.

Mindfulness is fundamental to the wisdom of the Buddha. In fact, the word *Buddha* itself means "one who is awake," one who is mindful. The rest of us, who are awake only at times, are part-time Buddhas. Though there are many people who have moments of clarity and mindfulness, a true Buddha is one who is this way continually, moment after moment. The more awake you are, the more you can melt frozen behavior patterns that keep you stuck in repetitive, negative cycles.

The Threshold of Pleasure

Drugs prevent you from enjoying the simple things in life. One way they do this is by raising the threshold of pleasure. Drug use is such a strong stimulation that, compared to it, other experiences pale. In the case of opiates such as heroin or morphine, your brain already produces similar chemicals of its own, called endorphins and enkephalins, but in minute quantities. An injection of heroin delivers massive amounts of a similar chemical to the brain. Compared to that, the small dose you receive from natural experiences seems insignificant.

Once you get used to this artificial, massive invasion of chemicals, it becomes difficult to notice the milder pleasure of everyday things like the natural high of exercising or seeing a sunset. By comparison, these experiences seem puny and piddling. You have raised the bar of what counts for you as a pleasure so high that no normal life experience even registers.

Mindfulness, on the other hand, is the exact opposite. Mindfulness is about opening to the subtle things, the exact shade of green of a tree, a child's smile, the taste of the morning air when you step outside to pick up your newspaper. Mindfulness lowers the threshold so that you can pay attention again to smaller pleasures and natural highs. It is a little like coming to appreciate subtly spiced foods after eating food full of hot chili. When you're used to hot chili, oregano seems like kids' stuff. It may not even seem to have much taste at all. Tuning in to normal life after the intensity of addiction is learning to appreciate subtler textures, tastes, and flavors. It is learning to appreciate the quieter intricacies of a Bach fugue after the pounding rhythms of acid rock.

To begin to come into the present and enjoy these subtler flavors, thinking about it is insufficient. Intellectual understanding, while important, is just the beginning of change. It is not enough. Deep and lasting change requires a direct experience, a new perception.

Untying the Knots

Mindfulness allows you to enjoy the life you have, instead of always fantasizing about having some other life. It allows the richness of each moment to unfold in a mind that is softer, more receptive. Enjoying the life you have, you find the energy to be more present also with what hurts. You begin to untie knots that previously seemed permanent. You find your way out of the binds of addiction.

The free-flowing awareness of mindfulness also issues in appropriate, effective action. For appropriate action flows from clear awareness. You cannot begin to take appropriate action on a problem until you see it clearly. When you increase your awareness of what is actually going on, you start to see creative, constructive, previously unimagined possibilities.

Returning to Now

One means for returning to the present is the practice of conscious breathing. Breathing is the most fundamental act of being alive. It is always available to you. To return to your breathing is to return to yourself, to leave the world of phantasms and fears, of useless conditioning and endless inner chatter and worry, and to come back to your true self. Breathing helps you calm the storm and be present with what is going on without running from it.

This practice is the foundation for all that follows.

PRACTICE

Be Aware of Your Breathing

Sit or lie comfortably. Notice where you are—what is going on around you. Be aware of your feelings from the events of your day. Now gently turn your mind toward your breathing. Do not interfere with your breathing. Just notice. Notice how your diaphragm expands and contracts, as if there were a small balloon in your belly. Allow tension in this area to dissipate. Just experience the breath. In and out. In and out. When thoughts pull you back toward planning what you are going to do next, worrying, or whatever, do not struggle against them. Just notice them. And gently come back to your breath. Notice what it feels like to breathe in. Notice what it feels like to breathe out. It is not a matter of thinking about the experience of breathing, but of feeling it, sensing it. Notice the inflection point, the point at which breathing in switches to breathing out. Notice also the natural pause between breaths. You do not have to decide when to breathe again. Your body knows by itself.

Normally we do not think of breathing as anything special; it is just breathing. But when you actually experience breathing consciously, it can be very pleasant and refreshing. When you do breath awareness correctly, it is a delight.

When you turn back to reading or whatever else you are doing, notice the subtle effect of having spent a few moments with your breathing. Try to spend moments on this whenever you can throughout the day. For example:

- while you are waiting in traffic or at a red light
- while you are waiting in line at the bank or the grocery store
- when you have finished one task and pause before you start the next one
- while you are waiting for your partner to get ready to go out
- when the television program pauses for a commercial
- while you are waiting for your computer to boot up

See how many other moments you can find to practice breath awareness during the day.

Urges: Handle with Care

Becoming more mindful is directly helpful to the process of recovery. For example, one of the challenges everyone trying to stop an addiction faces is that, from time to time, urges surface. These can be triggered by inner states, such as disturbing thoughts and emotions, hunger or tiredness, or by cues in the environment, such as driving past the house of a friend you used to drink with. Urges can be powerful, overwhelming desires—"I've got to have a drink *now*!"—or a subtle and vague discomfort, a barely noticeable blip on the screen of awareness—"There's something I used to do in situations like this . . ."

When we ask people in therapy about urges, they often want to deny them. To admit to an urge can seem like admitting a weakness, or admitting that somehow recovery isn't working. This is fear-based thinking. Actually, however, the key to urges is mindfulness. Urges will come and go, like any other thought or feeling. It is not this coming and going that is the problem, but the fear you attach to these thoughts and feelings. Fear makes the thought sticky, attaching you to it, causing you to lose your mindfulness. Instead of bringing mindfulness to the thought and embracing it, when you are afraid, you lose yourself in the thought.

An urge is a signal: something is wrong, out of balance. There's something in your life that needs attention. It is like an alarm clock going off, telling you it's time to wake up. But whereas in the past you thought it was the alarm clock that was the problem, and you just turned it off and went on sleeping, now you must remember that the sound of the alarm serves a purpose, even if it is not a pleasant experience. Instead of shutting it off, listen. Wake up!

To handle urges effectively, you have to first let yourself be aware of them. You cannot deal with something you do not first acknowledge. With mindfulness, you come to see that urges only exist for a limited period of time. You learn to view them for what they are: passing phenomena, just like all other thoughts and feelings.

The trick, then, is to become aware of the urge. Once you are aware, you have choices that were not possible when you were unaware. A woman Beverly worked with did nonstop household chores in the first few days of being smoke free. When her house was finally immaculate, and there were no more chores left to do, she actually created busywork by emptying dresser drawers that were already neat and organized, simply to create the task of refolding clothes. Reaching the point where you can take such steps, however, requires enough mindfulness to know that an urge is present.

If you practice breath awareness, you become used to the idea of thoughts and feelings coming and going without having to bother much about them. Breathing in and out, you can watch the coming and going of urges in the same way that it is possible to be present with anger and not be violent, or act out any other difficult thoughts or feelings. Or you can decide to give your attention to some task or other in order to navigate through the period of the urge.

"I'm Supposed to Breathe!": Anne's Story

Anne has been learning the practice of conscious breathing. Three months ago, she quit smoking and has been doing quite well with it. But Wednesday was a bad day. It seemed like everybody in the office was in a positively gloomy, sullen mood. So was Anne.

It started early that morning. In the shower, she dropped the bar of soap right on the most sensitive part of her instep, causing her to howl in pain. She forgot to put water in the coffeemaker, and ended up missing her morning coffee. Already late when she left the house, she hurriedly drove the three blocks to the freeway, only to come to a sudden halt once she got on it, as three lanes of traffic funneled into one because of road repairs.

When Anne took a phone message for her boss, she got the return number wrong. Despite the fact that it was someone her boss knew well and whose phone number was easily accessible on her boss's Rolodex, Anne was called on the carpet for this mistake—way beyond what was appropriate. Suddenly, Anne felt a powerful urge. "I could handle this," she told herself, "if I could just have a cigarette." Anne stepped outside where she used to smoke. Being there made the feelings even stronger, but then Anne remembered that there was something she was supposed to do in this situation. "Oh yes," she thought. "I'm supposed to *breathe*." She identified what she was experiencing as a relapse urge, and decided to distract herself from it by going for a walk. Outside, she focused on the many positive elements of her immediate experience: the pleasant sensation of her muscles working in harmony, the feel of her feet gently caressing the earth with each step, the blueness of the sky, the pleasure of each deep breath of fresh air. In twenty minutes, the urge had vanished.

Facing Life

Anne used smoking to avoid facing life problems, to escape for a while. But while this helped in the short run, in the long term it only strengthened a pattern of avoidance, of not being where she is. It is painful at times to look at what is and be present with it, whether "what is" means uncomfortable feelings, or a sense that one has had enough of something that brings pleasure. Because of this, we seek distraction, diversion, entertainment, or some sort of project—anything to move away from the painful awareness that what is is not what we want it to be. One person may deal with this pain through heroin, another through gin, still another through cocaine. If the concept of addiction is expanded to include excessive behaviors in general, some may seek relief through work, sex, television, or food.

When we become more open to what is, we are less compelled to escape reality in destructive ways. If alcoholics and others who are addicted are individuals who seek unawareness of difficulties, what happens when they learn to pay more direct attention to their bodies and minds? What happens when they stop their war against what is? What if alcoholics learn some of the ancient disciplines of awareness such as meditation, hatha yoga, or contemplative prayer?

Research on Transcendental Meditation has demonstrated that as people learn to manage stress through meditation, the desire for and use of drugs decreases. This suggests that such disciplines can help some people meet an underlying spiritual need, and thereby not only aid recovery, but facilitate growth. What if individuals who drink too much, for example, or eat too much, were taught to proceed more slowly with these activities, to taste every sip or bite fully, to feel the effect on their bodies and minds? Could this be helpful? What if people with such problems learned to pay close attention to how they feel, emotionally and physically? Approaches such as Vipassana meditation, journaling, or insight-oriented psychotherapy can all play a part in this. Such approaches may be especially powerful as part of an overall philosophy and approach to life, and not just an add-on or technique.

Drugs Don't Have the Magic—You Do

Countless media messages have hypnotized us to expect drinking to make us happier, more sociable, and more sexual. However, there is a body of research that teases apart what alcohol really does from the power of psychological expectancy. This research demonstrates that alcohol *in itself* does none of the positive things we expect. It has these effects solely because we *expect* it to have these effects, because these effects are part of the story we tell ourselves about alcohol. In itself, alcohol is a depressant drug. The pharmacological effects of depressant drugs are the opposite of many of our myths and expectations. Far from making us happy, outgoing, and sexy, depressant drugs actually make us morose, withdrawn, socially inept, and boorish. And they *interfere* with sexual functioning. Of course, we all think we know how drugs and alcohol affect us. But the power of psychological expectancy in drug effects is so profound that in at least one scientific study, marijuana smokers felt no effect from marijuana until they were in a social setting that provided cues about what they were *supposed* to feel.

Another example of myths about what drugs do concerns the comparison between heroin and alcohol. Heroin is thought of as a serious drug, alcohol as a more tame, domesticated drug. In fact, alcohol is seldom acknowledged as a drug at all. And so we say "drugs and alcohol" as if the word *drugs* did not include alcohol. Because of these attitudes, it is generally assumed that heroin withdrawal is an intense and serious matter, while withdrawal from alcohol is minor. The exact opposite is the case. Heroin withdrawal has been described as like a bad case of the flu—uncomfortable and unpleasant to be sure, but not resulting in any permanent harm. Alcohol withdrawal, on the other hand, can be life threatening, and must often be medically managed.

The powerful effect of drug expectancies on the body is well known. Medical studies routinely give some participants sugar pills or placebos when testing the effectiveness of new drugs. To be considered effective, a treatment drug must not only be more effective than no drug at all, but also more effective than a "fake" drug. While this is normally thought of as just good experimental procedure, it also shows the power of expectancy. Because of this power, some positive effect is always found for sugar pills alone. Sugar pills may be the miracle cure of all time, having at least some positive effect on virtually every kind of human disease and problem.

In actuality, of course, the magic is not in the sugar pill, nor is it in the alcohol or the cocaine. *The magic is in ourselves*, if we can learn to tap it directly.

PRACTICE

Reclaim the Magic

Take out a piece of paper and a pen or pencil. Close your eyes, and gently focus on your breath. Feel each inbreath, feel each outbreath. Enjoy this basic process of being alive for a few moments.

Consider the magical expectations you have about any drug or compulsive habit, and where these expectations came from. What is your myth about how this thing affects you? Where did you learn it? Note these things down.

Turn every expectation about a drug into an affirmation of yourself. For example, if you are thinking of alcohol, and your myth is that alcohol makes you sociable, tell yourself, "The power to be sociable is in me." Say this quietly to yourself, coordinating your words with a few outbreaths. Remember times when you have felt sociable without alcohol. If you are thinking that cocaine makes you feel sexual, remind yourself with the outbreath, "The power to be sexual is in me." Imagine yourself feeling very sexy.

Take back your own magic—the magic you have so carelessly given away.

Filling the Emptiness

When you stop using your drug of choice, there is a hole in your life where the drug used to be. Suddenly you are left with empty hours that you don't quite know what to do with. You try to do more of the things you used to do, but the activities you normally filled the hours with are now unable to meet the new level of demand placed on them. Often this is complicated further by the many problems that drug abuse leaves in its wake. The task before you at this point is to fill the void, just when things are at low ebb.

The almost overwhelming tendency is to try to fill the void with entertainment of one kind or another. And to a certain extent, this can be a useful strategy—at least in the short run—so long as the entertainment you engage in is healthy. However, this very tendency to try to fill every gap in life with something entertaining can ultimately leave you prone to return to addiction. For if you are in the habit of filling every minute with entertainment, there remains a risk that next time you might choose the entertainment of your drug of choice. What is needed is a different tactic: *A better way than trying to fill all your moments is to become aware of the fullness that each moment already offers.*

The experience of driving or doing the dishes or doing whatever you are doing is softened and expanded by this here-and-now, non-goal-oriented awareness. Such moments of awareness are moments of Buddhahood. If you can learn to multiply these moments, there is no need to attempt to enhance them through substance abuse. If you are trying to abstain from a drug and you are more satisfied and happy without it, you are not in much danger of relapse. But if you feel less satisfied, you are in great danger. Anything that increases your satisfaction with things as they are, that stops your personal war against reality, is helpful. There is nothing so dependably satisfying as being present with and enjoying the everyday. The everyday is sacred. By increasing your satisfaction with daily living in a healthy way, you become less prone to relapse.

PRACTICE

Establish Moments of Mindfulness

The ultimate goal is to be able to live mindfully all day long. In practice, however, this can be an overwhelming thing to set out to do all at once. When you try to do more than you are ready to do, you often end up accomplishing nothing except feeling frustrated.

One way to deal with this is to establish "moments of mindfulness"—parts of your daily routine that you set apart as times to practice mindfulness. Just as Buddhist master Thich Nhat Hanh talks about doing the dishes this way, so here are some other areas of daily living for which you may want to mentally set aside moments of mindfulness:

- taking a shower
- brushing your teeth
- making coffee or tea
- folding laundry

- preparing meals
- playing with your children

A shower, for example, is a great opportunity to be aware and enjoy what is happening in the present moment. You can tune in to the many pleasant sensations: the warmth of the water, the contact with your physical being, the sounds, the fragrance of the soap, the sense of being away from other things and having a few moments to yourself. Unfortunately, we often miss the opportunity to enjoy our shower in this way because we are occupied with our plans, worries, and fears.

We suggest you start with only one moment of mindfulness. Allow yourself a little extra time for this activity. Make it a time of peace. Be aware of your breathing. When you find yourself moving ahead to what you will do next, or dwelling on something in the past, gently come back to the present. In this way, daily activities that were neutral or even annoying can be turned into moments of being awake, aware, and alive. You can realize that you are happy and that you have no toothache. That is, you can become aware of the many things that are right. Then, when you are able to do this one thing in a mindful way, you may want to add another area to your moments of mindfulness. Choose one of the above, or invent one for yourself.

All the Everyday Things

Normally, we all think of hope as a good thing. And Beverly and I agree that it can be. It is pleasant to have things to look forward to. But Buddhism teaches that hope is a problem. How can this be?

Hope can be a problem if you are counting so much on things in the future that you are not alive in the present moment. If you wake up in the morning, and all you are doing is hoping to get through the day until work is over, you miss a lot of living in the meantime. If you keep postponing your life until that vacation or other special event, you never live *now*. Worse still, even when you get to that vacation time, you are still looking forward to something else, or focusing on the ways in which it does not live up to your expectations.

Sometimes the problem is that we count too much on things going a certain way. "I will be happy if I can earn more money, lose some weight, get the right career, find the perfect relationship." These are all wonderful things, to be sure. Yet when we ride any particular aspect of life too hard, we are doomed to disappointment. In the screenplay of the western *Lonesome Dove*, Gus McCrae, a cowboy Buddha, is talking to Laurie. Laurie is heartbroken because she is set on going to San Francisco and this does not seem likely to happen. Gus tells her: "Laurie, listen to me, listen to me now, pretty little thing. You see life in San Francisco is still just life. If you want only one thing too much, it's likely to turn out a disappointment. Now the only healthy way to live as I see it is to learn to like all the little everyday things."

Life in San Francisco is still just life. Life with whatever it is we now desire, that we hope will make us happy, is still just life. Only a life that takes joy in the little things of the present moment is a life of peace, happiness, and fulfillment.

PRACTICE

Stop Making Hope an Obstacle

Many times we think we cannot be happy until we get to some San Francisco of the mind. Perhaps you think that you cannot be happy until you are in a relationship, or leave one that is no longer good for you. Or you imagine you cannot be happy until you increase your income or finish your degree. The problem is that life with a good relationship and life with more money and life with a degree is still just life. Of course these can be good things. But even with them, you still have to get out of bed in the morning. You still have to struggle with the problems inherent in being alive.

Get out a piece of blank paper, and close your eyes for a moment. Tune in to the experience of your breath. At the top of the page, write the following:

"I will be happy when . . ." Then begin to write down whatever occurs to you.

When you are done, look over what you have written. Ask yourself, How can I stop using these as obstacles to enjoying my life as it is now? How can I tune in to the positives of my current life situation?

Enough

Moderation is an issue many of us struggle with. Some people may be prone to excess because they lack the internal recognition to know when they have had enough—enough to drink, for example. There are those fortunate people who do not have this problem and reach a point where they simply lose interest in drinking more alcohol. For them, it is not a moral struggle, but a sense of just not *wanting* any more alcohol. They are aware of the signals that say, "Enough!"

Abstinence does an end run around this lack of an internal gauge for having had enough. If you stay away from alcohol altogether, then there is no problem about not knowing when you have had enough. Other approaches have evolved to compensate for this lack of internal awareness. These include things like setting specific goals and keeping records of consumption. For example, a problem drinker may set a limit of two drinks per episode, no more than one per hour, and no more than six total in a particular week. Keeping accurate records provides an external structure to monitor consumption, which compensates for the lack of internal awareness. Support groups provide an external structure of a sort as well—in this case, a social one. For one thing, if you're at an AA meeting, you're not at a bar. For another, such groups provide support for abstinence and social consequences for relapse.

Awareness is important in all areas of excess. If you eat too much ice cream, watch too much television, or work too much, you are not living mindfully. If you are mindful, the first few spoons of ice cream, perhaps the first television show, the first task accomplished, may bring delight. But if you pay attention, this begins to change. At some point, you find yourself continuing something you no longer even enjoy because you have the *idea* that you are supposed to enjoy it. But your *experience* is otherwise. For this reason it is vitally important to get at the direct experience itself and not just the idea of it.

PRACTICE

Recognize Enough

Devote at least one day to mindfulness of when you have had enough of something, and as much as practically possible, stop that activity when you reach that point. This can include noticing:

- when you have had enough to eat
- when you have had enough to drink
- when you have had enough exercise
- when you have had enough sleep
- when you have seen enough television
- when you have done enough work
- when you have had enough time alone
- when you have had enough time with others

The idea is to tune in to your own organism and, as much as possible, respect its limits. As a teaching by negative example, Beverly and I recently completely exhausted ourselves planting our vegetable garden. In one day, we rototilled, raked, added fertilizer and peat moss, and planted. For people unused to such labor, this was way too much for one day. Blisters and fatigue put us out of harmony in body and mind for the next day or two. What did we gain by pushing so hard? We had let the external goal of finishing the garden take over all other considerations, including the most basic consideration of all—a harmonious life.

Instead, for at least a day, let the standard be your own harmony and well-being. Do enough. Then stop. You be the center, the judge. Do not be pulled away from your own well-being by external considerations of any kind. As the ancient sage Lao-tzu has taught us, just do enough, without striving and struggling.

Of Garbage and Sunsets

Mindfulness is everyone's birthright, as natural as drawing breath. At first, children reveal a startling capacity for fresh, novel perception. They find as much fascinated delight in the garbage heap as in the rainbow. And this persists until the world teaches them what they are *supposed* to notice, what they are *allowed* to comment on. Gradually children learn to call the garbage heap ugly and the sunset beautiful.

And gradually the things they say come to reflect a shift toward what adults consider more appropriate objects of attention.

To become mindful involves a return to the fresh and direct perception we knew as children. That is why Jesus taught that "unless you turn and become like children, you will never enter the kingdom of heaven." Mindfulness involves the art of being childlike, without being childish.

A character in the film *American Beauty* loves to use his video camera. One of his favorite pieces of video is several minutes of a plastic shopping bag swirling and dancing in the wind. If you look with unprejudiced eyes, it is extraordinarily beautiful. But if you are caught in your categories of thought, you only see a piece of garbage. Mindfulness allows you to see many wonderful things with fresh eyes, beyond classifying your experience into what you like and don't like.

By the time you became an adult, the process of alienation from your own perceptions can have gone quite far, including your emotions. I once led a men's therapy group in which members of the group told one member that he was angry. This man actually stood up, shook his clenched fist, and yelled, "Damn it! I am *not* angry!" This is a surprisingly common experience for therapists. Yet in subtle and not so subtle ways, most of us are like the angry man, lacking full awareness or mindfulness.

Mindfulness reverses the process. Mindfulness is knowing when you are angry, and instead of trying not to be angry, becoming one with the anger. It is about taking care of your anger so it does not cause trouble. It is also about being present with what is really happening. It is exactly the opposite of addiction, since the addictive impulse is to deny what is going on when you dislike it.

The Miracle of the Ordinary

Mindfulness is not about tuning in to the remarkable and the fabulous. Seeking the remarkable and the fabulous is part of what traps us in addiction to begin with. Instead, it is about finding what has been called "ordinary magic." In a famous Buddhist text, the Buddha said, "I obtained not the least thing from unexcelled, complete awakening, and for this very reason it is called 'unexcelled, complete awakening.'" We keep looking for something outside of ourselves, outside our own experience, to have the answer. But we overlook what is right here at hand. We continually overlook the real miracle—the simple, startling fact of our human life and awareness. At first this may seem too ordinary and commonplace to bother with. But it is the source of the power we give over to drugs, the power we need to reclaim.

Approach mindfulness gently. It cannot be forced. You can create conditions that encourage enlightened awareness. But it is not helpful to be too goal oriented. Forget for the time being that you are trying to get anywhere or fix anything. Forget trying to become a Buddha. You are already a Buddha. Relax into just being. Paradoxically, the "passivity" of non-goal-oriented awareness in the here and now helps you to make active choices that shape a more positive future. This is a better understanding of the word *karma*, often misunderstood to be a kind of fatalism. Karma means that the deeds of today, if rooted in a clear awareness or mindfulness, create a happier future. You come to see what is *really* effective for you concerning work or career, health habits, leisure activities, relationships, and so forth, because you are no longer entranced by what you think is *supposed* to work.

Please experiment *mindfully* with the ideas in this book, paying attention to what works and does not work for you. You may find some thoughts and practices that are helpful to you on your journey. Remember that, ultimately, you must connect with the same source of wisdom that books come from. Our aim is simply to help you reconnect with that which you already have and already are.

It is common for self-help books to promise the moon. This is in actuality an apt expression, reminiscent of the Zen phrase "a finger pointing at the moon." Zen teachings are not the moon itself, but only the finger that points. It is the moon that is important. It is your own direct experience that counts.

Go out and take a look at the moon.

Doorway Two
TELLING LIFE STORIES

Whether I shall turn out to be the hero of my own life, or whether that station will be held by anybody else, these pages must show.

—Charles Dickens, *David Copperfield* (1850)

❧

Consider your life as a story you are still writing. Many people hold on to life scripts connected to their addiction, which perpetuate negative life stories as well as continued attraction to drugs and alcohol. You don't have to get stuck there. You can write a new story.

❧

A Story about Stories

Once a student asked a rabbi why God created human beings. Before you hear the rabbi's answer, pause to appreciate the question. For as is often the case, the question itself is the thing, and you won't appreciate the answer if you have not struggled with it. Put yourself in the teacher's shoes for a moment. How would you answer? Why did God create human beings?

There is an understanding behind the question that God, abstractly considered, is complete in himself.* And because he is complete in himself and lacking nothing, why should he bother? In the Creation story in the first chapter of Genesis, God speaks, and light emerges. God speaks, and land is separated from water. God speaks, and plants, animals, and, in the end, human beings leap into existence. Human beings arrive last, the crowning glory of it all. But why should an eternal God, lacking nothing, full and complete in himself, do such a thing? Why should he bother?

What the rabbi said was quite wonderful. He said God created us *because he loves stories.*

If you believe in a God who is, as some theologians have said, "Wholly Other," this answer is nonsense. From a certain perspective it even makes God a sadist. For all of our suffering and struggling and dying is then a kind of divine soap opera told for the amusement of a remote and uncaring deity, a god who laughs at his creatures for worshipping him despite all the suffering he puts them through.

However, seen from the point of view that we are not separate from the Divine, then this answer is ultimately not about God, but about ourselves. And *we* are the ones who love stories. Since the time when our earliest ancestors gathered around ancient fires to reenact the successful hunt, we have loved stories. The tendency to view our lives as drama, as both tragedy and comedy, is so much a part of our nature that the only real question is what kind of a story we are telling with our lives, not whether we are telling one. Some stories are constructive, some are destructive. Some are satisfying, some are not satisfying.

Story and Beyond

Ultimately, the goal of mindfulness is to transcend story and make direct contact with the real. In leaving story behind, however, we may experience an emptiness akin to despair. Yet such despair may be closely connected to enlightenment. One Tibetan rinpoche, when

---

*We employ the traditional male pronoun, without subscribing to the concept of the deity being any particular gender.

asked what enlightenment was like, responded that it was the last disappointment of his life. At the top of his illustration of the mystic mountain, Saint John of the Cross wrote the Spanish word *Nada* (Nothing—which is also *Todo*, Everything). An anonymous mystic from the late Middle Ages referred to the highest experience of God as entering a "Cloud of Unknowing." Zen Buddhists aim at getting beyond words and concepts to direct, simple experience. All these are hints that, while we may need to be aware of our life stories and channel them in more positive directions, the ultimate goal is a leap beyond them, right through the very heart of despair into that fertile emptiness that is God, or Tao, or the Universe—the Ineffable Ground of Being. Ultimately, enlightenment is about letting go of all of our drama and melodrama, all of the little soap opera plots and subplots of our lives, and entering into the realm of just being.

This does not mean we become inhuman, however. And because it is human to tell stories, even the most enlightened people will think in terms of story, and teach in terms of story, and experience their lives as story. But they also have at the same time a quality of freedom from story. The Zen attitude is captured in the account of a student monk who wept upon the news of the death of a close relative. When a fellow student criticized this display of attachment, he replied: "Don't be stupid! I weep because I want to weep."

This account reveals someone who has by no means lost his sensitivity to life and life story. For it is not as though the highest virtue of Buddhahood is to be insensate, like a rock or a hunk of metal. But there is a certain freedom from story, not being entirely caught up in its net of illusion.

In the meanwhile, however, there is no escaping the fact that we are storytelling beings. The way is not to try to avoid this, but rather to see it all the way through. If we are ultimately to develop a certain freedom from the limitations of a narrative point of view, we must first become mindful of the stories we are telling.

Storytelling

Storytelling is an essential human quality. In this chapter, we examine the stories we tell ourselves about who we are. What are these stories based on: truth, fiction, what our parents told us, what our first-grade teacher said, or what our neighbors led us to believe? Perhaps the stories we hold were once adequate but are now outdated or too one-sided. Growth is a process of telling more adequate, comprehensive stories about who we are until we develop the freedom to go beyond them.

In this chapter we examine the connection between life story and substance abuse. By examining these stories, we help you uncover some of the myths that block your road to recovery. What do we tell ourselves about the food and drink we take into our bodies? How do we glamorize our stories, telling tall tales, and mythologizing what we consume? Perhaps it is time to edit a well-worn life story of who you are and how you want to spend the precious opportunity that is human life.

The human tendency to tell stories is pervasive. Even scientific theories, which tend to be thought of as something quite different from story, are themselves a kind of story we tell about the way things are. To be an adequate scientific story, a story must meet certain criteria and serve certain purposes.

But perhaps our most important stories concern ourselves and who we are—whether we are beautiful or ugly, successful or unlucky, even whether we are mechanically inclined or artistic. These personal stories intersect with our stories about drugs, both the fables we have about how drugs affect us as well as our legends about what kind of people use drugs. To change negative habits, it helps to appreciate these underlying meanings.

Looking at Your Life

What kind of story are you telling with your life? Is it a healing story? Is it a story of glittering success and accomplishment? Or is it a story of pain and shattering failure? Is it a story of being liked and respected? Or one of being ignored and avoided? Are you writing a story about yourself as a creative person? A problem solver? Or someone who is helpless and can't deal with life? Is your story line about a person who is kind and caring? Or about someone who is selfish and hard? Are you someone who is mechanically inclined? Or a klutz? A mindful person is aware of these story lines, and learns to use them in a fluid and flowing way, rather than be caught in them rigidly.

A prison inmate told Beverly a life story of being a superbly expert car thief. He boasted of perfecting the art of stealing cars so that he was able to break into and start any car within ten seconds. He delivered his story complete with police chases and miraculous getaways, often just in the nick of time. His Billy the Kid self-image was an absurd, but intact, life story.

Beverly gently suggested an alternative. She pointed out that he actually must not be very good at being a car thief. After all, he had been caught and arrested for the third time. Perhaps he should find another life pursuit. He agreed that this was true, but argued that he had analyzed his past mistakes and had plans to refine his technique for future thefts. He was convinced that next time, he would be unstoppable. His life story of the perfect car thief was a myth he was not ready to change.

The car thief's story may seem to contain obvious traps, distortions, and fallacies. But the problems in our own stories are not always so easy for us to see.

PRACTICE

Write Your Own Obituary

First sit quietly. Breathe gently in and out. Think about your life. Let the images and memories come freely, spontaneously, without trying to control their content. Take your time and don't be in a rush. Then write an ideal obituary for yourself— the one you would like to have written about you. Return to quietness, breathing gently in and out. Then write the shadow-side obituary, the one you would most hate to have written, but which you fear contains a grain of truth. Now examine the two and consider the differences. Is your ideal a reasonable one, or is it so inhuman as to all but guarantee frustration? Is it *too* reachable, or is your ideal not high enough? There may be no easy answers, but the most important thing is to hold the question in awareness without forcing an answer. The feared obituary can give you some clues about what gets in the way, about your shadow or inferior side. How realistic are these fears? Can you recognize your own features, albeit distorted, in the ideal obit? In the feared one?

Beverly and I have not yet encountered anyone who said he wished he had spent more time working or had earned more money. And we have never encountered anyone who said she regretted spending so much time with people she cared about.

The Magic of Eating and Drinking

Simple actions such as eating and drinking, as well as drug use, have many levels of meaning. Some of these meanings are evident in religious ritual. Eating and drinking are not only about survival, but these are also symbolic actions. When we eat and drink, we feed on life. We are participating in the basic process by which life transforms life into other life. There is no escaping this. Even the strictest vegan feeds on living things. When we drink water, we kill countless microorganisms. By eating, we transform the life of plants and other animals into human life.

In this way, by eating and drinking, we participate in what is perhaps the most basic mystery of life itself. The Jewish Passover celebration demonstrates an understanding of this by making special food and drink a means of connecting with the story of God's deliverance of the Hebrews out of Egyptian bondage. Jesus built on this foundation by establishing the ritual of Communion as the central rite of Christianity, telling his followers to eat the bread as his body and drink the wine as his blood.

There is magic here. In fact, the phrase "hocus pocus" originates in the Latin words of the priest (*hoc est corpus meum*, this is my Body) that transform the Eucharistic elements. And indeed it *is* magic. By the process of eating, we take lettuce and beef, chicken and green beans, and *hocus pocus!*—transform them into human life: human bodies, human action, human awareness, human loving and hating, dancing, killing, praying, creating, thinking, feeling, pondering, remembering, anticipating—all manner of human being and human doing. Ultimately, eating and drinking are acts full of mystery. They are God taking God into God.

We do not need religious ritual to be aware of the transformative magic of eating and drinking. In fact, if we were more deeply aware of it—if we could see how the universe is contained in a slice of ordinary bread—we would need nothing more. But most of us have become so estranged from the wonder of eating that we look to ingest things that seem more exciting and potent. When we cut ourselves off from the wonder of the everyday, from a view of our lives as a meaningful story rather than "a tale told by an idiot, full of sound and fury, signifying nothing," it is no wonder we try to fill ourselves with the artificial, ersatz magic of drugs. When we are alive to the wonders of ordinary eating and drinking and ordinary life in general, we no longer need chemical enhancement of them.

Our Estrangement from Story

So what happened? How did we become estranged from the story-telling language of spirit? Part of what happened is this: We desperately attempted to become modern people, people of science rather than people of myth, legend, story, and religion. And we very much needed to if we were to get past burning witches and torturing people with different religious views. Yet this has created a deep split in our psyches, for our fundamental nature as storytellers has not changed. We still need stories. Dangerously, these things have been relegated to the unconscious, where they control our fate all the more. Part of the problem of overeating and overdrinking is precisely that these acts have been sterilized, disconnected from the fabric of larger meanings to which they nonetheless belong. The Old Testament says that the God Yahweh is a "jealous god." For gods that are forgotten, that are not given their due, become vengeful. Greek mythology is likewise full of accounts of the human troubles that ensue when gods and god-desses feel neglected. From our modern perspective, we look at all this as silly. But the meaning is clear: When we deny spiritual significance and meaning, we pay a horrible price. Not because God is some sort of evil potentate, a kind of Big Meany in the sky who demands attention. But because we cannot deny what we are. We are divine beings. We are composed of the energy of the stars. We are creatures of myth and legend and story, far more so than creatures of logic and rationality. And while we cannot and should not attempt to enter this realm with the literalism of our ancestors, denying its importance costs dearly.

In *Man and His Symbols* (1964), Swiss psychologist Carl Jung expressed this modern dilemma:

> Modern man does not understand how much his "rationalism" (which has destroyed his capacity to respond to numinous symbols and ideas) has put him at the mercy of the psychic "underworld." He has freed himself from "superstition" (or so he believes), but in the process he has lost his spiritual values to a positively dangerous degree. This moral and spiritual tradition has disintegrated, and he is now paying the price for this break-up in world-wide disorientation and dissociation.

Story and Addiction

Profound human change this side of enlightenment occurs through changing our life story. It is for this reason that we cannot just change by deciding to change, but must come to view ourselves in a different way. If your underlying story says that you cannot succeed, then until that changes, no matter how you push yourself, there will always be something holding you back from success as if by some mysterious force.

The stories we tell ourselves about addictions often differ sharply from medical and scientific fact. And in a way, these differences are actually the most interesting parts of our stories, because they show so clearly that it is story that is at work rather than pharmacology.

Story and Alcohol

Alcohol makes us sexy. Alcohol makes us happy. Alcohol allows us to be more sociable, less inhibited, more outgoing and fun-loving. When we drink, we are the beautiful people, the successful, the famous, the fast-driving, hard-hitting, James Bond types. If we have troubles, alcohol allows us to forget them for a while. We can feel wise, free and easy when we get a little intoxicated. And of course, if we feel this good when we get a little intoxicated, won't we feel even better when we get more intoxicated? An ingredient in this underlying myth is that more is always better. And if more is better, then we naturally feel deprived if we encounter limits or are advised to abstain.

Prison inmates bragged to Beverly about their alcoholic escapades. Most of them, when challenged, would begrudgingly admit that alcohol or drugs helped land them in prison. One inmate told of heading straight for the liquor store upon his previous release from prison. He reported a hazy recollection of the event, but was re-arrested for wielding a gun on a city bus and wildly shooting straight up through the top of the bus. He was unaware that a destructive myth about alcohol continued to be his undoing.

The reality of alcohol is quite different from our stories about it. It makes us socially boorish, stupid, unable to function sexually, less able to do things requiring coordination and quick reaction times like driving a car, let alone driving fast and well. The reason we believe it does wonderful things is that we have entered a different realm when we drink: the realm of story. Our story or expectation about alcohol endows it with the properties of a magic potion. And these expectations override its actual, chemical effects. If the fault is in ourselves and not our stars, the magic we think alcohol releases is in us as well, and is strong enough to overcome the actual effects of alcohol through our belief in its enchanted powers.

Other Drugs

The stories we tell ourselves about drugs besides alcohol are similar and are told for similar reasons. One of the properties of stimulant drugs, for example, is that we feel powerful and wonderful when we take them. However, as with alcohol, not all of our experiences from stimulants are the actual result of the drug. Stories of people rubbing their sexual organs with cocaine because this is a sexy drug, for example, make no sense at all scientifically. This only makes sense from a mythic perspective, seeing cocaine as a magical substance that gives us great mana, or power. In reality, however, cocaine is a close cousin of novocaine—the drug your dentist uses to numb your mouth. And like its relative, cocaine decreases both sensitivity and blood flow. Neither of these effects are really desirable properties for sexual functioning. And while we may think, as with alcohol, that we become splendid and witty conversationalists under the influence of stimulants, that is not how others experience the stimulant user.

And what about the drugs that do the opposite of stimulants, that make us feel calm or euphoric? Marijuana, barbiturates, and heroin are examples. The sensations are pleasant. Certainly, some of this is the drug itself. But how much of it is that, for the time being, we have simply become insensitive to the pain of our lives? In a way, this is probably the *main effect of all drugs of abuse: to desensitize us to our life problems*. If we could experience both the effects of drugs and the consequences of their use more objectively, we might be a great deal less tempted by them. But we are tempted because they make us less sensitive to our environment, less aware of the painful gap between how we would like our lives to be and how they actually are. This in itself is euphoric in the way that you feel light when you lay down a heavy backpack that you've carried for miles.

The other major class of drugs of abuse is the hallucinogens. This class of drugs includes LSD, peyote, and mescaline, to name a few. Interestingly, this is the class of drugs that has been the most tempting to spiritual pioneers, feeling that these substances connect us to the realm of our deeper nature, the place in us from which myth and legend originate, from which comes the sense of the Presence of God. Perhaps these arguments have some merit. We do not want to exclude the possibility that these substances may have a spiritual use, as they are employed by shamans and native healers, for instance. At the same time, while the allure of such substances reveals a deep, human hunger for direct, living spiritual experience, this hunger can be fed more safely and less brutally by other means.

Drugs and the Rebellion Story

Of course, individual reactions to drugs will vary. There are physiological differences in how people react to and metabolize a drug. And individuals will have different reactions based on what kind of particular story or meaning the drug has for them. But there are some common, identifiable themes.

One very common theme in drug use, including alcohol, is rebellion. If drug use is related to rebelling against parents, for example, this may well shape the person's experience of the drug, making it seem more exciting. For those in committed relationships, it may function as a rebellion against a controlling partner. Illegal substances probably always involve some rebellion, in this case against society itself. Illegal drug use crosses a line as minors who drink cross a line also. However, it is quite a different thing to do something that is permitted by society, although for adults only, than to do something that society prohibits for everyone. Teenage drinking, as an act of rebellion, involves a component of being grown up, of coming of age. Ironically, this means that one of the reasons young people drink to excess is precisely that we forbid them to and reserve drinking for adults. But using a substance that society says is illegal for everyone goes further still, placing the user well outside the mainstream.

Drugs and Outlaws

For at least some of us, drug use involves the theme of being an outlaw. Curiously, being outside of the law in the United States is not always viewed negatively. It is different in countries where people are more compliant with authority. But here, outlaws are a kind of hero. From Billy the Kid to Jesse James, from Bonnie and Clyde to Robin Hood (whom we have adopted as our own from English legend), the idea of being an outlaw taps into feelings of romance and freedom. It also underscores our ambivalence about law and authority, and our fear of the limits these may impose.

Outlaw myths are powerful and peculiarly American. They shape not only drug use but also such related problems as gangs, whose members see themselves as outlaws. The outlaw myth is particularly powerful in the American psyche because it compensates for our conscious view of ourselves as always good and benevolent, the self-giving saviors of the world. Yet the shadow side, the less pure and altruistic side of ourselves, must be expressed. We allow for this at least in a partial way through outlaw legends. Even then, of course, it is a very partial expression, and our outlaws must generally find themselves outside of the law for good reason, the victims of compelling external circumstance. Thus in the classic Hollywood outlaw western, the protagonist becomes an outlaw through a set of perfectly understandable, totally exonerating circumstances. Robin Hood is a thief, but this is excusable because he is redistributing wealth to the poor.

The reality is strikingly different from the myth. Real outlaws are not beautiful people. They inflict horrible suffering and misery. Recently a young man and woman were arrested in Colorado after going on a cross-country killing spree that began in New Jersey. The reality of this horror show was quite possibly obscured for these young killers through an identification with the outlaw myth. One can understand why the ancient Greeks described such psychological states as being in the grip of a dai-mon or a god. For most of us, it is one thing to romanticize Jesse James, and quite another to put a gun to the head of a living and breathing human being and pull the trigger. But if you are deep enough in the clutches of an outlaw myth, you can numb yourself to these realities.

For many the experience of using drugs is colored by themes of being grown up (if the person is young), being free (in fact in some cases, being so free that the law does not apply anymore), being pow-erful, being sexy, having fun, being an adventurer, being special and not just one of the masses, and so on. The more "out there" the drug, the more it may connect in particular to the outlaw myth. Thus heroin, crack, and LSD are a lot more "out there" than marijuana or valium, and involve greater rebellion.

Of course, identifying these themes is not sufficient for change. For the story itself is the thing. And abstract discussion will not move us nearly so much as watching a good old movie glorifying the exploits of Frank and Jesse James. Some individuals, for one reason or another, have failed to find positive life stories and themes with which they can identify. In part, this reflects the vacuity of roles available in our success-oriented culture. For such people, the outlaw and rebel themes, as well as other negative life stories, are powerfully compelling. They are compelling because the real *terror* is not whether your life story is positive or negative, but not having one at all. Not having a life story confronts us with the void, with emptiness, with meaninglessness. Using drugs not only temporarily numbs pain, but also supplies an alternative meaning. One can see oneself as an outlaw and rebel, as a kind of modern Billy the Kid. Or you can even see yourself as simply a failure and a washout. Some story is better than no story at all.

Ask yourself how much this theme has played a part in your attitude toward drugs and alcohol. If there is a need to feel more free, a need to rebel, which most of us have to some extent, it is not necessarily the best thing to try to suppress this. Are there more positive, creative ways to express this need? Maybe you need a black leather jacket; maybe you need a motorcycle. Maybe you need to blast your rock'n'roll now and again. Or maybe you could get involved with constructive social movements. For example, people involved in environmental protest may also be operating out of a rebel or outlaw myth to some extent. Only they are doing it in a way that connects them to the circle of life rather than cutting them off from it.

PRACTICE

Claim Your Freedom

Place a pen and some writing paper in front of you. Sit quietly. Close your eyes. Take long, deep breaths, slowly in and out. Clear your mind before beginning this exercise.

Imagine your mind as a clear, blue, open sky. Whatever thoughts and feelings come along are like clouds or birds going past. They appear and leave, but do not affect the basic openness and freedom of the sky at all.

After at least several minutes, open your eyes, pick up your pen, and begin listing the things that help you feel free.

Recovery Stories: Sin and Redemption

Stories of recovering from drug dependence, especially within the framework of Twelve-Step programs, have a common structure. These are stories of sin and redemption. One way to try to recapture a redemptive moment is to recall in horrifying detail what preceded it—namely, the sin. This is why people at Twelve-Step meetings recount the awful things they did before they started the program. The effect of this, hopefully, is to strengthen the decision to change, to stay sober. But there is a risk.

If one has truly left old ways behind, and built a meaningful, satisfying life, these stories at some point lose their compelling power, or worse still, they keep one trapped at an earlier stage. This danger is reflected in the common Twelve-Step emphasis on always being "in recovery," never recovered. Perhaps this encourages vigilance, but it may also keep a person stuck. Mental health advocates would protest in horror if we talked this way about other psychological diagnoses, and appropriately so. To forever label someone who has had a depressive episode as a "recovering depressive" or as "depressed but in remission" does not build on strength, but rather perpetuates a negative life story.

Working in a residential treatment facility for adolescents, Beverly quickly found that these teenagers were acutely aware of what was supposed to happen in substance-abuse groups. The group participants began taking turns telling their "I fell so far down that I did this" story. It was clear that their response was mostly pro forma, and did not run very deep. It wasn't until she established a more human connection that they shared things about themselves outside this rigid structure.

Confessional stories told by rote are not helpful. One aspect of such stories is the reliance on something or someone outside of oneself to bring the redemption. In other words, no redemption without a redeemer. For some this is God. For others, it may be the group itself. However, this is not the only way to see things.

PRACTICE

Weigh the Pros and Cons of Sin/Redemption

Like all stories, the story of sin and redemption can function in both positive and negative ways in your life. Consider how relying on a Higher Power has helped you at times. In what ways has it been helpful to let go of control and trust it all to Grace? Then consider the flip side: where would it have helped more to rely on your own insight and ability? Has there been any rebounding between the extreme states of sin and redemption, between being on and off the wagon? Record your insights.

An Alternative: The Hero

For some people, and maybe for all people at some times, other types of underlying myths are more helpful. What about the myth of the hero, for example? Hero myths are quite a different type of story. A journey is undertaken. Trials are endured. Perhaps some of the gods are on your side, but others are neutral or even opposing. By all of this struggle, the hero is transformed and transfigured. And in the end, there is a triumphant homecoming, a victorious return. In its optimism and self-reliance, this is a much more fundamentally American myth, and perhaps a more fundamentally Western myth in general. For we, after all, think of ourselves as the explorers, the wilderness tamers, the self-made men and women, the independent thinkers. The ubiquitous bumper stickers WHY BE NORMAL? and QUESTION AUTHORITY show these themes to be still powerfully present.

The hero story emphasizes the theme of self-reliance. A related psychological term is *internal locus of control*. An internal locus of control is a sense that life is what we make it more than accidents that befall us. People with an internal locus of control show less evidence of psychopathology than people with an external locus of control.

This paradigm is quite different from the sin/redemption sequence. In essence, it says: "I was really caught up in drugs. I used them for many years. This cost me important jobs, important relationships, and almost my life. But in the end, I pulled myself out of it. It took several attempts, and a few times I think I tried to fool myself without really changing. But in the end I did it. Some people helped me with advice and support. But I really did it myself. I discovered a strength within that I didn't know I had. And now my life is better, and I am a different, better person for the ordeal. For I know I have the strength to pull myself out of negative habits and patterns when I need to."

This is the very sort of story that tends to be associated with enduring change. Psychotherapy outcome research, for example, has shown that people who attribute change to the therapy or the therapist tend to relapse, whereas people who see their own efforts as the cause of improvement maintain therapeutic gains. Therefore, successful clients may say something like, "I liked talking to Tom, and he really seemed to understand me. But I made the changes myself."

Both types of stories have been useful to people recovering from addictions. But because of the dominance of the Twelve Steps, only the first type—sin/redemption—is officially sanctioned. Hero stories are generally whispered more quietly, not proclaimed at the meeting. Yet these stories emphasize values of individual strength and self-reliance, which many would find more helpful and congruent with how they feel about themselves.

A root question behind this, too, is whether the God/Redeemer is out there, or, as mystical traditions generally teach, within. Sometimes it is comforting and helpful to think of God as out there, a Divine Someone whom we can pray to, turn to in crisis. But if God is out there, then so is Evil. If we are saved by external divine forces, we can be damned by external evil as well. None of this tends to foster a sense of responsibility for one's life. But if God is within, not as the individual persona or ego, but as the Ground of our Being, then we also have to deal with our own evil, our own shadow side. This theme is reflected, for example, in the *Star Wars* series, when the hero, Luke Skywalker, must face one last challenge to become a true Jedi knight. He must face the evil, the dark side of the Force, in the guise of his own father, Darth Vader. That is to say, he must face the evil in himself.

In Buddhist practice, one takes refuge daily in the Buddha. Part of what this means is to take refuge in the Buddha within, that aspect of ourselves that is already wise, awake, and enlightened. This is a variation on the hero theme—hero as enlightened person. Perhaps it will be more helpful to some people to touch that part of themselves that is already a Buddha or a Christ than to continue to focus on past mistakes.

Negative and Positive Life Stories

In sum, the life stories of people who are addicted to a drug contain themes of power, rebellion, or being a special person who is above the rules—that is, an outlaw. Often people with drug issues have a profound ambivalence about authority. These themes may also sometimes be embedded in more general negative stories of failure and inadequacy, of alienation and not belonging. Different types of emotional problems may reflect a predominance of one or more types of life themes, as drug use seems to be related to rebellion, for example.

When you consider how deeply drug use is tied to story and myth, the absurdity of Nancy Reagan's "Just say no" slogan, and of Bob Dole's "Just don't do it," becomes clear. Not only do these statements ignore the vast differences of subcultural forces, of poverty and negative role models and hopelessness and abuse, of the difference between an advantaged upper-middle-class suburban teen and a minority ghetto child, but these slogans ignore the fundamental propensity of human beings to view their lives as story. Simple, direct approaches can help with a few people. But persistent problems do not yield so easily because they connect with deep life themes. Perhaps this is why so many of us have had the experience of trying to force a change in our behavior in one way or another only to find it extremely difficult.

Direct approaches and slogans may serve a purpose in marking the accepted limits. They draw the line and enjoin us not to cross it. But these approaches also perpetuate the problem. Such slogans make people who identify with drug subcultures, and who have life themes that have incorporated this fact, feel all the more outside the mainstream, all the more different and alienated. And feeling more alienated, it becomes far easier to say, "Oh what the hell. . . ."

At least part of what is at issue in changing human attitudes is the spiritual question of how to come to see oneself in terms of a more positive life story. How can we come to see ourselves, as Dickens asks, as the heroes of our own lives, rather than as failures and outcasts?

PRACTICE

Contact the Hero Within

Sit comfortably in a straight-backed chair or on a meditation cushion. Close your eyes. Take long, slow, deep breaths. Let your mind wander back in time, letting yourself remember times when you did things that you felt good about, moments when you had a positive sense of who you are. If any negative thoughts come up for you, don't fight them. Simply let them float away. Include scenes of childhood triumph: the day you scored the highest in the class, the time you hit it out of the park, the day that attractive person agreed to go out with you. Remember also your adult triumphs: the day your work obtained some recognition, the time you got a raise, moments when you felt a deep and powerful concern for others. Refrain from minimizing your virtuous actions. You have positively impacted other people's lives. Take it in. When you are ready, open your eyes.

Our Stories and Religion

Religion helps us identify with a larger story, of which our individual stories are a part. Each of us must appropriate the story individually if these collective stories are to be meaningful. Otherwise, they are empty. Religion attempts this appropriation through ritual. For example, a Twelve-Step group member may see herself as part of the ongoing Twelve-Step story. But to appropriate this collective story effectively, her individual story must mesh with it. If your individual story is negative in theme, it may be difficult to see yourself as part of a positive tradition.

Another problem is that some of the old stories are not as compelling to everyone as they once were. Some themes in the Judeo-Christian story are now quite strange to modern ears. To understand God as a king, you have to enter the worldview of the ancient Middle East. In that view, the world consists of a group of smaller and larger potentates. And God, in such a world, is of course the biggest potentate of all. This is very alien to a society in which elected presidents are considered popular with a sixty-percent approval rating. Appreciating the ancient view of things can involve some rather serious mental contortions.

The point is not that the old traditions cannot be interpreted in more meaningful ways. They surely can be. But to do so, you must let it interact creatively with modern culture and with your own basic myths. Caution is in order to ensure that old traditions do not serve to intensify negative individual stories. For there is always the danger that the old ideas can be assimilated into a negative narrative about your own life rather than become a source of peace and strength. This can happen when, for example, a person of low self-esteem accepts all too easily that he is a sinner, accepting this as a psychological reality rather than a theological one. A narcissist connecting with Eastern traditions that emphasize God within, on the other hand, can all too easily see himself as God. This is not always helpful, either.

The Story of Enlightenment

Enlightenment, too, is a story. It is a story in the sense that it expresses a deep truth, and like all stories that are deeply true, it calls us onward, evoking a sense that peace is possible, that joy is possible. Once you leave behind the negative stories that have kept you trapped in your addiction, and you start to see your life in terms of more positive stories, the lure of the story of enlightenment may pull you toward a state that is ultimately beyond story altogether.

Yet to say that enlightenment is a story is also true in the sense of being "just" a story. This is why Zen teacher Shunryu Suzuki said there is no enlightenment, but only enlightened activity. In this sense, it is important to remember that enlightenment is nothing other than clear, calm, moment-to-moment awareness. We miss it when we think of enlightenment as only some grand experience or exalted psychological state. The true enlightenment lies concealed in the wondrously ordinary. It is concealed, that is, in the same way that the fish does not know the water it swims in or the bird the air it flies in.

Changing the Story of Your Life

Your basic life story can be changed. Yet certainly you cannot just decide to invent a more positive story, snap your fingers, and have it be so. To try to do this in some superficial, overly rational way is like the tail wagging the dog. But through processes that enhance your awareness of which stories are being played out and when, and perhaps with the help of a therapist or wise person at some points, you can over time change your story in profound ways.

In the next Doorway chapter, we will introduce journaling as a mindfulness tool that can also help you be more aware of your story. But if you desire to free yourself from identification with a destructive life story, it is imperative to remember that your story has been in place for some time already. It is unkind to expect change overnight; expecting too much too soon keeps you trapped in a negative view of yourself. Think of change as a marathon, not a sprint. It is more like growing, the way a tree grows toward the light, than like constructing a building. Give yourself time. This work requires patience with yourself and a gentle persistence, not sudden and muscular bursts of effort. Approach the change process with calmness, not desperation.

Doorway Three
JOURNALING

Listen to your life. See it for the fathomless mystery that it is.
In the boredom and pain of it no less than in the excitement
and gladness: touch, taste, smell your way to the holy and
hidden heart of it because in the last analysis all moments are
key moments, and life itself is grace.
—Frederick Buechner, *Now and Then* (1983)

✦

*Use journaling to deepen awareness of your life story and open the
door to spiritual awakening. Regular journaling brings the power of
mindfulness to bear on repetitive problems and aids in contacting
your inner wisdom.*

✦

In the throes of addiction, we feel as though our drug is our only
friend. When strong emotions and life difficulties hit us hard, we
have only one practice for attempting to contain these feelings:
using our drug. In this sense, it does not matter whether we smoke,
drink, or shoot heroin. All are equal. All are attempts to contain our
troubling emotions.

It is important to notice that there is a positive, healing intention behind substance abuse. We are looking for a way to bring some healing and peace to our troubled minds. We are not using because we are bad people trying to do a destructive thing. We are using because we are trying to do something good, *but in the wrong way.*

What are you to do then, when you make a commitment not to follow the path of substance use anymore? How are you to stick to your intention when strong emotion drags you down? The false friend substance abuse may have revealed itself for the fiend it really is, but you still need a vehicle to contain difficult feelings and bring healing awareness to them. You need something to prevent you from losing perspective or drifting in the flood of feeling.

There are many practices that can help. There are many things that can initiate a process of healing. Sometimes another person can help, especially if it is someone who has some mindfulness, some peace and stability. Such a person might be a family member, a teacher, a therapist, or a friend. But since no one can always be available, you need a friend who is always available, someone who can always give you deep listening. There is such a friend. That friend is your journal.

The journal can seem overly simple, just as breath awareness in meditation can seem overly simple. But do not be misled. The Buddha taught that breath awareness can bring us all the way to enlightenment. From one point of view, likewise, a journal may seem to be just sheets of paper. But these sheets of paper contain a universe of healing and help. They are no less than a master teacher, who brings you back to the zone of mindfulness.

The Policeman May Be a Bodhisattva: Sarah's Story

A series of things had gone wrong that day. Sarah had quit smoking five months ago. It was tough going in the first weeks. She was anxious and irritable most of the time, and could think of little else but lighting up. But gradually—very gradually—these feelings waned. She had started practicing breath awareness regularly, and had come a ways in establishing some stability. Most days now, she could sit quietly for fifteen or twenty minutes, and smile and enjoy her breathing. In fact, as things piled up on her today, Sarah had continued to practice, breathing in and out with her worry and struggle, watering seeds of calmness in herself.

But then on her way home from work, she glanced in her rearview mirror and noticed a police car. "He couldn't be after me," Sarah thought. "I'm not speeding." She jumped as the siren startled her out of her reverie.

He told her she had run a stop sign, and she knew this was probably so, because indeed she did not recall seeing a stop sign. She felt terrible. The officer's cold, authoritative demeanor triggered powerful feelings of badness and shame in her. She accused herself of failing in her mindfulness practice for both missing the stop sign and letting these feelings overwhelm her.

By the time Sarah got home, she felt a hair's breadth from going out to get a cigarette and light up. She tried to practice breath awareness for a little while, but it was difficult in her present state. It helped a little, but the negative thoughts and feelings were still too strong in her. She was still in danger of relapse: she was still suffering. Then she decided to open her journal.

Sarah took her journal out slowly, mindfully. She had been writing in her journal now nearly every day for a week, and had established a positive atmosphere around journaling. She opened to a new page, wrote the date slowly, and then wrote down the word *Beloved*—her way of addressing the Divine. Sarah felt that when she wrote in her journal, she was speaking directly to the heart of God.

Breathing in and out, writing slowly and thoughtfully, she let her thoughts and feelings pour onto the paper. She took care to be next to her feelings of shame and sadness and anger, trying not to get lost or stuck in them on the one hand, or deny them on the other. She noticed each thought and feeling with loving, gentle attention, knowing herself to be more than these thoughts and feelings. When she reached a place where it felt right to stop, she did so.

Now Sarah switched gears. She paused, breathing in and out, listening—listening for that still small voice within. Then she recorded what she heard. She heard many things. She heard that the policeman was a bodhisattva. She had been in a state of nonmindfulness, and she had been driving dangerously. The Universe sent him to jolt her out of it, to force her to slow down. Sarah now saw that, while the experience was not enjoyable, it protected her from worse possibilities. There were other insights as well.

By the time Sarah was done writing, she felt much better. She had contacted the wise part of herself, and put the struggles of the day into a more positive framework. She was back, centered, aware, her true self once again. Later in the evening, the urges came back again, along with some of the painful feelings. But she now found that she could work with them. By containing her feelings in her journal, Sarah was able to transform them into something manageable. She was all right.

Reaching the Wisdom Within

Too often, we look for wisdom outside of ourselves. We run to the bookstore to read the latest spiritual teachings available in print. We attend retreats and workshops. We go into therapy. And all of these are good things; all of these can be helpful and immensely valuable. But ultimately, any external source of help is there to aid you in contacting your own inner wisdom. That is its true purpose. If you use it to foster an addiction to external sources of wisdom, it will lead you astray.

Even when Buddhists go to a dharma talk, a talk given by a Buddhist teacher, what they are doing psychologically is contacting their own inner Buddha. They are not listening for new information, but for the source of all wisdom, that which lies behind all words and teachings. They project their inner Buddha onto this teacher. And if he or she is a worthy vessel for that projection, the teacher helps the listeners touch the Buddha in their own hearts. It is for this reason that teachings are important. We do not read or hear talks ultimately to add to our academic knowledge, our store of show-off information. It does not truly matter if you can recite the Three Dharma Seals or the Four Establishments of Mindfulness, or quote chapter and verse from scripture. The purpose of these things is solely to put you in touch with the God within. And it is for this reason that journaling is such a powerful practice.

Swami Vivekananda, a disciple of Ramakrishna and a powerful teacher in his own right, expressed this in his own characteristically dramatic way: "Books are useless to us until our own book opens; then all other books are good so far as they confirm our book. . . . We are the living books, and books are but the words we have spoken. Everything is the living God, the living Christ; see it as such. Read man, he is the living poem. We are the light that illumines all the Bibles and Christs and Buddhas that ever were. Without that, these would be dead to us, not living" (Swami Vivekananda *Meditation and Its Methods*, 1946).

This is what Sarah was doing with her journal, and it is what you can do with yours. Your journal is the book you use to transcend books, to go straight to the source from which all true books come.

PRACTICE

Learn to Write without Censoring

Think of a minor issue that has been on your mind. At first, avoid anything as major as an impending divorce or a move to another state. Instead, choose a topic that is of some importance to you, but not a life-altering issue. It could be something like whether to befriend a new neighbor, which charity to make a contribution to, or perhaps whether to enlarge the family room.

Choose your topic and sit comfortably with a pen and paper ready. Set a timer for five minutes. Pick up your pen and start writing. Write anything and everything that comes to mind about the topic you chose. Don't censor anything and don't stop writing. Free-associate from one thought to the next. This is not an exercise in journaling yet. It's an exercise to help you get comfortable writing your thoughts down on paper. Do not try to construct grammatically correct sentences, and do not cross anything out. Just write. Write until the timer sounds.

Chemistry of the Soul

When we think of alchemy, many of us think of poor deluded souls who were trying to turn base metals into gold. In his pioneering work, psychologist Carl Jung showed us that alchemy has a deeper meaning. Jung demonstrated that, while as chemists or manipulators of matter the alchemists were unsuccessful, their work nonetheless tells a great deal about psychological or spiritual transformation. Their rich and complex symbols may not have revealed much about the physical world. As *chemists*, their work was off track. But as students of the chemistry of the soul, they revealed a great deal about human nature.

The alchemists typically would combine all manner of secret substances into a *vas*, or vessel, place a lid on it to contain the substances, then apply heat. And as is generally the case when something is cooked by intense heat, the substances did not remain the same. They changed and transformed. The first thing that would happen was called the *nigredo*, or darkening. The heated substances would turn black and foul. But this blackening was the essential first step of transformation. Without it, it would not have been possible to produce the gold or philosopher's stone that was the goal.

Jung saw in this a deep psychological fact about human growth and transformation. The *nigredo* in human life is usually triggered by some challenge. Insofar as our point of view is limited, distorted, or one-sided, life will throw us a curve at some point—a curve that we can only handle if we submit to the painful darkening, the dark night of the soul that precedes all awakening. This is a horrible, painful, disorienting crisis of some kind. For some, addiction can be just such a crisis, and just such a prelude to transformation and change.

Think of your journal, then, as just such an alchemical *vas*. It is a container in which you place the raw elements of your experience, the problems of living that you encounter. You hold them in this vessel, and apply the heat of your awareness or mindfulness. If you are unwise, you may consider the raw materials of your everyday experience and struggle as garbage, as junk to get rid of as soon as possible so you can become a spiritual person. But such an attempt to avoid life always has consequences. Spiritual practice must not be a way of avoiding life, as drug abuse is. If you use your spiritual practice in that way, you will have substituted one problem for another. Rather, spiritual practice is about *transformation*. It is about taking the raw material of daily life and transforming it into wisdom, peace, and joy. The negative elements in life are at least as important as the positive ones in the process. Leaving them out vitiates your transformation process.

Choosing a Vessel

If you are ready to begin journaling, you must first choose the actual notebook that you will write in. If you think of this as being a vessel of transformation, you may want to do this carefully, mindfully, tapping your intuitive sense of what feels right. Just as the alchemist of old would carefully choose a vessel that could withstand the heat, that was strong and would not crack, so also it is helpful to be selective in choosing the book that you will write in. Bookstores and office supply stores these days contain many attractive unruled volumes for this purpose. You might like to approach your journey to the store as a kind of ritual. Don't do other errands on the way; don't look at other items in the store. But make this trip especially for the purpose of obtaining your vessel. As you stand before a selection of journals to consider, breathe in and out. Find one that speaks to you, that feels like a good container, that inspires peace and confidence and positive feelings. Buy it and bring it home.

Keep It Private

What do you think would happen to an alchemist who chose a vessel that leaked? What would happen if he kept taking the lid off while heating the contents? Obviously, the result would be very unsatisfactory. There would be little chance of deep transformation if that were the case. For the function of a container is to *contain*.

For this reason, it is very important that your journal be kept *private*. If you do not keep the process private, elements will keep leaking out that will prevent the transformation. If your journal is not private, you will be aware of that fact when you write, and it will not feel safe to record the raw feelings and thoughts and experiences that you want to make a space for. We make the same recommendation about therapy to therapy clients and for the same reason, asking them to consider the therapy room a sacred space, protecting what happens there even from the person the client is closest to in all the world.

For this reason, it is a good practice to keep your journal in a safe place. Do not leave it open on the kitchen table, for example. If you do that, you have only yourself to blame should someone read it. Tell the people you live with that you expect your journal to be respected as private, and do your best to explain why. Explain that it is to their advantage as well. Think of what would happen if you were to have a fight with your partner and you had not told her about your need to keep your journal private. You practice sitting meditation and walking meditation, and you want a safe place to contain your angry thoughts and feelings. So you write in your journal. You let the pain spill out, then you try to hear the voice of God within, helping you see things in perspective. Later your partner reads the section where you are spilling out your pain. And it waters seeds of pain in her. Perhaps your partner does not even get to the part where you are attempting to reach a higher perspective on the problem, but only reads the angry things you wrote. If this happens, you have only compounded the trouble. But if your partner respects the sacred space of your journal, then you are free to work on transforming your anger before you speak with her again. If your partner allows this space, it will be to her advantage, because you will be a transformed person rather than an angry one. You will be able to approach your partner with greater calm, love, and wisdom, and she will be protected from the toxin of your raw anger.

Of course, it is perfectly all right if you select a passage to share out of your journal, just as you might select one or two things to share about your therapy session. But reporting everything blocks deep transformation. Deep transformation requires a safe space, a sacred space. It requires a certain solitude. If you do not respect your own solitude enough to protect it, it will not be deep enough to help.

Starting to Write

When you begin to write in your journal, take it carefully from the place where it rests to the table or desk where you will work. Do your best to let this be a place of peace and solitude. If it is unavoidable to be around others, ask their cooperation when you are writing in your journal. Just as you would not like to be interrupted while you are meditating, you do not want to be interrupted while writing in your journal. Turn the phone off or put the answering machine on. Just as you have selected your vessel carefully, you might enjoy having a special pen for your journaling. The special notebook you selected, the special pen, the special place of peace all contribute to your contacting the special place of peace and wisdom within.

It is helpful to begin writing on a new, fresh sheet of paper each time. Write the date at the top. You might like to spend a few moments breathing in and out consciously. Perhaps you will want to say a prayer of intention, such as, "May this be for my healing, and for the healing of all beings"—or whatever form of prayer puts you in a receptive frame of mind. Then see if an area of concern emerges. Is there something in your relationship you are concerned about? Is there a problem at work? A question about how to parent your children? A worry about finances? Is there some important decision you're facing? See what comes up. Sometimes you might know immediately what you want to write about. That is often the reason you pick up your journal in the first place. At other times, you might like to let all of your major life issues surface, briefly enumerating them before choosing the one of most concern at this time. Then let the concern pour out of you.

A word of caution: even as you are letting the concern pour out of you, remember that it is not helpful simply to rehearse negative things. It is one of the destructive myths of pop psychology that ventilating raw feelings is good in itself. Being in touch with negative feelings is only helpful if you can bring some peace and mindfulness to them. So even as you let the feelings and thoughts come out on the paper, practice breathing in and out. Be in the present moment. Be aware of the feel of pen and paper and the flow of ink onto the page; enjoy the physical act of writing. Try to breathe and maintain some sense of calm awareness about your feelings, neither stifling the feelings nor losing yourself in them. If you feel more angry or upset when you are done writing than when you began, chances are you are losing yourself in the emotion. You may need to step back a little from it. On the other hand, if you feel cold and cerebral as you write, and have a kind of bottled-up feeling when you finish writing, you have probably not allowed your feelings to flow freely enough. Buddhist texts talk about mindfulness of the body *in the body*, and mindfulness of feelings *in the feelings*. This means that you must not be removed from your feelings, but in them. In the moment that you have a feeling, it and you are the same. When you are angry, you are your anger. There is no separation between you and your anger. Yet if you get lost in your feeling, forgetting that you are also more than your feeling, this will not be helpful. That is not mindfulness. Mindfulness is a balance.

The Still, Small Voice

Once you have written out your concern, allowing it some space, some loving attention, you might like to take an additional step. That additional step is to contact your own inner wisdom, the voice of God within.

In the biblical story of the prophet Elijah (I Kings 19), the prophet went out into the wilderness in despair at the apostasy of the people of Israel. Standing on a mountain before God, a mighty wind came, powerful enough to split rock. But God was not in the wind. The wind was followed by other mighty phenomena—an earthquake, and a fire. But God was not to be found in either of these. Then there came a still, small voice. And it was in the still, small voice that Elijah heard God. And God empowered him to leave the desert of his despair and reenter life.

That still, small voice is available in our time also—not just to great prophets, but also to you. It is more powerful than what seems to be powerful, more powerful than wind and earthquake and fire. If you become quiet and still enough, you can hear that voice. And it will send you back into your life with the power and strength you need.

You might be able to contact your wise inner voice without formal preparation. Just breathe in and out a few times, let God speak to you, and write what you hear. However, if this is a new practice for you, or if your concern is a large and difficult one, it might help to prepare a little. For example, you might wish to picture yourself as sitting before the feet of Christ. See him as clearly as you can; feel his presence. He has listened deeply, lovingly to your concern. Now he pauses, choosing his words, and speaks to you. Write down what you hear him saying to you. Or work with a shamanic image: see yourself entering deep into the earth through a special, sacred opening, and coming to a place of great holiness where you encounter your own wise inner self. Write down what you hear. Your preparation might be the utmost in simplicity, just a few conscious breaths, or an elaborate visualization—whatever helps you contact your inner wisdom. When you are done writing, pause, breathe a few conscious breaths, then read it over again slowly, drinking in the wisdom you have just contacted. Trust it.

You might be tempted to dismiss what you've written or tell yourself it is all just your imagination. Don't. It is only in recent times that we have become so dismissive of our imagination, making a contrast between it and the supposedly real. Imagination is a valuable spiritual capacity. It is a store of rich insight. Imagination unlocked the shape of the DNA molecule and took us to the moon. Imagination is the way we grasp truth, not just with our heads, but with our hearts. And besides, if you are just making it all up, pause to consider how you are doing that. Where are you making it up from?

So the final step is extremely important—having some faith in the wisdom you have contacted.

An Example

Perhaps it would help to see an example of what it might look like to conduct such an exercise. Here is a selection from my journal. It was written during a mindfulness day when I was aware of my wandering attention.

Sunday, Aug. 6, 2000

The Concern
I know I am transforming—becoming a much happier, more peaceful person. At the same time, I am very aware of how, at some point every day, I switch modes and lose mindfulness for a while. It's connected with an attitude of rushing forward to the next thing. There are so many little movements, gestures, in each task, which I approach as though doing them only to get to the next thing. For example, getting a cup of coffee. I approach it with mindfulness, aware of pouring, stirring, etc. But then I notice I closed the refrigerator door without awareness, just trying to get this little part over with! Similarly, shaving, showering, etc. There's such a strong habit energy pulling toward the future.

Or sometimes the pull manifests as a certain restlessness, a desire for entertainment. So yesterday, I wanted to see a movie, discovered it was showing shortly, and pushed everyone to go, getting caught up in fighting traffic and rushing so as not to be late. Mindfulness out the window!

How can I learn to slow down? How can I live one day in full mindfulness?

Inner Voice
First, you must not fight against yourself. This is very important. These habit energies are garbage, and the garbage is always a potential flower. Do not fight! Embrace these feelings with peace, awareness, understanding.

Second, learn to allow space. Every moment does not need to be filled with something, with some activity. When you stop trying to fill moments, you become aware of the underlying fullness already there.

Third, see if you can pause and come back to yourself the moment you discover you have been pulled off center. Try to stop everything else, meditate for a little while, return to yourself.

For we have all been sold a bill of goods—this feeling that somewhere there's something exciting going on, and we're missing it. As though there were a wonderful party going on, and you were not invited. As though you have to struggle to find that party and get yourself to it.

This never works; for when you get to the party, you are not present anyway. You have the feeling the real party must be somewhere else.

There is an irony. There *is* a party going on. But it is right here, right now, as close as your next breath. And you are always invited.

After writing this, I felt much better, and was able to pursue my practice of mindfulness more deeply.

Types of Concerns

I might just as well have chosen an entry about another kind of topic, but I chose this one because it was a good example of an answer from inner wisdom. But please do not imagine that legitimate concerns are only about your mindfulness practice and other spiritual matters. One of the flaws of much spiritual practice is that it divides our world up into good and bad concerns and issues. Issues of sexuality, money, work, relationships, not to mention relapse urges or slips—these are all very legitimate concerns. They are also very spiritual. Do not divide your life up into areas that are worthy of mindfulness and areas that are not.

A Perfect Life?

Sometimes you may not know what to write about. The mind sometimes resists our attempts to channel it in certain directions. So just because you have the intention of identifying and exploring a concern, your mind does not necessarily go along with the idea. Then you find yourself blocked.

Fortunately, you can work with this very property of the mind to get unstuck by working paradoxically—so-called reverse psychology. If you don't find a concern leaping out at you, sit and breathe consciously. Then tell yourself several times, "Everything in my life is perfect and wonderful just as it is." Try to make yourself believe this statement as the absolute truth. Usually this will be enough to trigger awareness of concerns. If it does not, you have a lot to be grateful for indeed.

Worries, Worries, Worries

Sometimes we are in a position of having far too many worries. This is often the case when we are new to mindfulness practice, so there is a backlog of areas needing awareness. This can also happen when we are living through a particularly difficult time, some dark night of the soul. Then concerns flood into our awareness all at once, each clamoring for our attention and healing awareness. Yet if you try to deal with them all at once, you will only add energy to feelings of desperation, and your journaling will not bring healing.

In this case, first list all your concerns, giving each one a short title or handle. Breathe in and out quietly and read the list over. See if one concern stands out as something you want to bring awareness to. This may be the concern that feels most pressing, but if that concern is also overwhelming to you right now, you might start with another one—one you feel a readiness to work with. Then work with just this one concern for now. Acknowledge the others and promise to revisit them at a later time. You do not have to try to address everything all at once.

What Inner Voice?

Sometimes it may happen that you know perfectly well what concern you want to address, but once you begin to listen for your voice of inner wisdom, you do not get an answer. There are several things to try.

First, breathe in and out consciously for a few minutes. Then read your concern over slowly, with deep awareness. Listen to this concern as you would to a concern of the person you loved the most in the whole world. See if this does not free your inner voice.

Second, try one of the visualizations described above or one of your own invention to imagine your inner guide in some definite way. Take some time with this. See this embodiment of inner wisdom in as detailed and concrete a way as possible. Envision his or her surroundings clearly. See if then perhaps your guide does not want to speak to you. If not, allow this to be okay. Perhaps it is enough, right now, just to hold this concern in mindfulness before this wise person.

These are not just empty words. Holding our issues up to the light of mindfulness—perhaps as here in the form of an inner guide who embodies the principle of mindfulness—is already a healing activity. In *The Way of Passion* (1994), Andrew Harvey tells the story of a woman who had lost everything, and sought out the wisdom of the Hindu saint Ramana Maharshi. She poured out her grief before him, but he was silent. Growing impatient, she chastised him for not offering words of wisdom or consolation. He remained silent. She then wept uncontrollably until, exhausted, she finally looked up into his eyes. In his eyes, in the silence, she found an inexpressible transmission. Harvey comments: "There are no solutions to life, but there is an experience of bliss, of being, of the deathlessness of the Divine Self, of Silence in all its multifaceted, diamond splendor that heals all grief, all wounds, all questions." This conclusion also applies to inner gurus who are not manifested externally.

Finally, given what was said above regarding the recalcitrant nature of the mind, you can try working in a paradoxical way. Breathe in and out and persuade yourself, "It is completely okay just to have brought mindfulness to this concern. I do not have to hear the inner voice today." The beauty of this approach is that it is completely true. Just the act of bringing mindfulness to an issue is already helpful, even though you may have to do this repeatedly with difficult life problems. So one of two things will happen, either of which is good: either you will see that it is okay not to get a specific answer this time, in which case you have done enough for now, or you will resist this message, and your inner wisdom will begin to speak. Of course, that is also okay.

Slips and Urges

As we have said, this book is not so much for people who are still struggling actively with addiction, though even there it might be of some help. It is more for people in the maintenance stage of change—for people who have quit, have established some stability in quitting, and are now seeking to stay quit by building a satisfying way of life and cultivating their spirituality. Nonetheless, we have known people who have not touched a drop of alcohol for many years who, upon being suddenly confronted by overwhelming loss or difficulty, have a powerful urge to drink again or even have a slip. It happens. A person who was once severely depressed, for example, has an increased risk of depression reoccurring. It is as though, once you know the way to the dark place, you can find your way back there more easily than those who never found it to begin with. If your dark place is substance abuse, there's a chance of your being confronted with this issue again.

Whether you have actually relapsed, or are just encountering an urge of some kind, mindfulness is your friend in dealing with this, too. When the relapse episode has ended, breathe in and out, and record your experience. Identify the triggers that caused this urge or relapse. Note them down. Identify everything that you are telling yourself, everything that you are aware of feeling about the urge or slip. Try to get beside all of these thoughts and feelings, embracing them with kind attention, but not losing yourself in them.

Many people will say life is a learning experience, but when we are having a difficulty, we do not want to pay attention. We do not want to learn. We want to run from the problem. Addiction is one of our culture's main ways of running. Mindfulness is the opposite of this impulse. If life is a learning experience, and everything we encounter a teaching, then why not do the learning? Let's see what we can learn about this experience, so hopefully—if it is a negative one—we will not need to repeat it. Did a difficulty ambush us emotionally, something we were not prepared to deal with? Or were we taken by surprise by an encounter with our drug of choice being all too easily available when we least expected it? If you have relapsed, ask your inner guide what you need now to get back on track. Ask what you will need to prevent a relapse in the future.

A Different Outlook

When you ask these questions and bring mindfulness to these issues, you have already begun to change your situation. For one thing, you have already switched from a passive orientation to a more active, problem-solving stance. This is already miraculous. When we talk to people at the beginning of substance-abuse treatment, there is often a lot of initial unawareness. Often, such individuals are unaware of their true thoughts and feelings. When we ask what led up to the slip, they do not have anything to say. "It just happened," they tell us. And that is indeed the way they experience it. It seems to have struck them like a thunderbolt out of a clear blue sky. "I was just walking down the street, when—*wham!*—suddenly I was in a bar drinking again."

The reason it feels that way is lack of mindfulness. So when you do something to bring mindfulness to the situation, the addictive process can no longer just run itself out on autopilot. Once you look more deeply, you see there are always things that lead up to significant urges or relapse. If you keep shining the sun of mindful awareness on the issue, the problem will eventually shift and yield. And what seemed impossible becomes easy.

You might want to be especially aware of the danger of black-and-white thinking in this regard. It is all too common in the addiction field to think in such terms: you are either on or off the wagon, either doing well or a hopeless case. You may have had months or years of success, but consider one day or even a few hours of relapse as incontrovertible proof you are nothing but a no-good addict. This is distorted and unrealistic. One slip does not undo all the good you have done with a period of success. Even a relatively short period of sobriety is a partial success. And seeing it that way will empower you to get back on track more quickly, with less pain and suffering both for yourself and those in your life. Shine the light of mindfulness on this distorted reasoning, and come back to yourself. Challenge the unrealistic, black-and-white thoughts.

PRACTICE

See Mistakes as Part of Living

To learn from a slip, get to a quiet place and open a notebook. Breathe. Let your mind wander lightly over the incident you are concerned about. Note any thoughts and feelings that occur to you. Notice the feelings in your body. Especially pay attention to what led up to the slip. What outer events played a role? What actions or words of other people were a factor? Even more importantly, what thoughts and feelings were triggered in you by these outer factors? Note all this down lovingly, giving yourself the understanding you might give a friend with a similar problem. Perhaps you made a mistake. You were not prepared to deal with this situation constructively. But avoid negative overgeneralizations or predictions such as "I'm no good," or "I'll never be able to change." Better still, if these thoughts and feelings arise, treat them the same as any other material. Note them. But contain them, rather than let them contain you. Don't get lost in these thoughts and feelings, but remember that you are larger than they are. There is more to you than these things. Allow yourself to experience such feelings, without giving in to them, without making them an occasion for further mistakes.

Guilt

It is helpful to notice the chains of doing, thinking, and feeling that lead up to a slip, so you can be prepared next time under similar circumstances. One thing leads to another, and another, and so on, until you get to the relapse. Jerry wants to stop overeating and lose weight. But today he got upset at work. As he fought rush-hour traffic on the way home, his turmoil grew. By the time he got home, he told himself, "I don't care, I'm going to eat that chocolate bar anyway. Hell with it." When Jerry reviews this in his journal, he touches all his thoughts and feelings about the incident. He notes them without judgment. He is curious. What made this situation so awful? What is the worst part of it? He notes shifts in his body, thoughts, and emotions as he writes.

By simply doing this, Jerry is already having a different experience. Normally, he would have gotten upset, and then gone on an eating binge. Later, guilt feelings would emerge. These feelings are painful, but avoiding them only ensures that he will not reexamine the pattern. That way, nothing changes. No learning takes place. The more he protests that he will never do it again, the more trapped he becomes. But by simply being with his experience with as much self-understanding and gentle acceptance as he can muster, Jerry begins to break the chains of conditioning that connect this inner turmoil with the addictive behavior.

If he can go a step further, he might ask himself how he might have handled this situation differently. He might reflect on how he could avoid this kind of situation in the future. Because Jerry has a tendency toward self-criticism, he must be cautious about the immediate urge to criticize the initial ideas that come to him. For sometimes we strangle our solutions before they are even born. Though some ideas might be better than others, he should first welcome all ideas equally. Later, after thinking of everything he could do to cope with such situations in the future, he can choose the ones that are most practical, that seem to have the best chance for success.

A Christmas Gift: Elizabeth's Story

If you journal about a relapse, it is important to look at the thoughts, feelings, and events that led to it, and identify alternatives. How else could you view the situation that triggered the relapse, and similar ones? What could you have done differently, said differently, thought differently?

Elizabeth has had a destructive drinking habit for five years. The problem grew slowly, perniciously, almost imperceptibly. By the time her drinking reached its peak, she had come to avoid social situations where she would not be guaranteed abundant access to alcohol. That meant she no longer socialized with people who were not heavy drinkers. They just didn't seem to be any fun. Gradually, her health deteriorated. An alert physician questioned her about her health habits. Elizabeth was startled to learn there were early signs of liver damage. A friend told her about AA, and she went to a few meetings. The views expressed in the meetings did not always fit her own experience, but she valued the support. So she kept going.

Elizabeth attended meetings regularly and was sober for three months. But Wednesday there was a bad winter storm, and the kids were home from school. Everyone was cooped up in the house. The kids were fighting and acting out. She blew up at them several times. She began to feel a powerful urge. "I could handle this if I only had a drink," she thought. Somehow this seemed entirely reasonable and rational. She tried valiantly to push the thought aside. But then she remembered that she still had one last stash. It was a bottle of Courvoisier she had received as a Christmas gift, and she just hadn't had the heart to throw it away. It was good stuff. At the time she had told herself, "I'll keep this for company." She never thought she would actually drink it herself. But today, when her oldest son, Sam, bloodied the nose of her youngest son, Darrell, she had had it. She told herself, "I just don't care anymore." She noted that the first drink didn't taste as good as she remembered. But she was past caring. Anyway, hadn't they taught her she was powerless to stop once she started? Her husband came home to find her passed out on the sofa and the kids running wild.

Elizabeth could use this incident to support a negative life story. She could tell herself that she was hopeless, incurable. But she could also make a different choice and tell a different story. She could learn to be with her negative thoughts and feelings, breathe gently in and out to calm them, and write about them in her journal lovingly and with self-compassion. She could also use her journaling to examine what she might do differently in the future. Virtually every aspect of her story suggests alternatives. Since she socialized almost exclusively with heavy drinkers, she might try to increase contact with non-drinkers or light drinkers. Since her health has been threatened, she might develop an overarching goal of cultivating greater health and well-being, for which abstinence is just a part of the answer. Such an approach would prevent focusing on drinking (or not drinking) itself, which sometimes only exacerbates the problem. Clearly she might have done something different with the liqueur. She might have challenged her idea of keeping the bottle for someone else to enjoy as setting up a relapse.

Elizabeth's journaling might help in many ways. She might reach a realization that she needs to learn to handle difficult situations with her children with greater skill. Is there someone who could give her a break from them for a while, trading child care time to allow some of the steam building up behind her ears to dissipate before it explodes? She could reexamine the myth that alcohol helps her cope. She might learn to challenge her thinking that a slip leads automatically to a fall. She might come to see, if she is aware of her experiencing, that the liqueur was not nearly so enjoyable in reality as she had built it up to be in her imagination, using this awareness to catch future slips earlier on.

About twenty minutes into journaling, Elizabeth began to reflect on the experience and consider solutions rather than remain stuck in the problem. At that precise moment, she turned an important corner. *As soon as we decide to do something to cope with a difficult situation, as soon as we decide to return to our mindful breathing and begin to transform our painful thoughts and feelings, our psychological state shifts from helplessness to empowerment.* That in itself makes a great difference. The slip becomes an opportunity to learn instead of additional evidence of her powerlessness and inability to change. She can see it as a situation she was not prepared to handle, one that requires new ways of coping, instead of the inevitable result of some relentless, incurable disease.

Gratitude Journaling

Psychology emphasizes the importance of not denying problems. It is felt to be supremely important to face your problems and issues squarely, to look them directly in the eye. But while psychology sees the danger of denial clearly, it misses another kind of danger almost completely: the danger of a negative focus.

It is true that problems must be faced. Mindfulness is a way of facing them, not like a gunslinger in some Wild West shootout, but calmly and kindly, lovingly and gently. But there is also a growing awareness in psychology of the importance of acknowledging positive things as well. Such a practice need not be a denial. Denial means denial of reality, but to deny positive elements in your life is just as much a denial of reality as to deny negative ones.

Our mental and emotional life is a garden. There is no such thing as a garden without weeds, no matter how well tended it is. There, alongside our lovely tomato plants, are those insidious little plants we do not want, but which grow so easily. It would be a mistake to ignore the weeds. They would overrun our garden in no time. But it is also distorted to see the weeds without seeing the tomato plants and lettuce and flowers that we want to grow.

Mindfulness puts us in touch with the world as it really is. We do not have to try to see things that are not there. We only need to open up to reality. Negative feelings such as sadness or fear have a way of narrowing our perception; positive feelings broaden it. When we are mindful, we see positive elements. Being in touch with these elements brings healing to the negative feelings. The effect of this on mind and body is often more profound than just taking care of the negative directly.

Many of us worry a great deal of the time. We focus on what is difficult and upsetting, on the problems we face, and we ignore the many good things around us. This is a distorted view, and requires strong medicine to counteract it.

One way to counteract a tendency to focus inordinately on the negative is to practice gratitude journaling. All you need to do is write at the top of the journal page, "Things I enjoyed today." Then list them. Be creative. See how many things you can identify that are enjoyable in your daily life. And of course, don't overlook small pleasures.

Negative experiences can deepen gratitude awareness. For example, Beverly and I recently had a plumbing leak, and had to have our water turned off for a day or so until the plumber could come. Ever since, we have been more grateful and more aware of having running water. Similarly, if your car does not work, you will be more appreciative of it after it is repaired; if you don't have the headache today that plagued you yesterday, you can experience the pleasure of no headache today.

Our friend Joe Boroughs likes to deepen awareness of the positive by focusing on some element in his life and telling himself, "I'd be happy if only I had *that* in my life!"—substituting something that he actually does have. You might enjoy trying this in your journal by writing, "I'd be happy if only I had . . . ," and then listing positive things that you do in fact already have. This will combat the tendency to focus on what is missing and remind you of the many good things that are present.

If you have a tendency to be somewhat focused on the negative, you might like to practice gratitude journaling for an intensive period of a few days or a week, perhaps returning to this practice periodically.

The Hero of Your Life

Every once in a while, it is helpful to look through your journal entries to gain perspective on the sweep and movement of your life over time. When you do this, you can look for themes, just as you might be aware of recurring themes in a novel. How does the protagonist in this novel—the novel of your life—seem to get into difficulty again and again? Can you see patterns? Can you see alternatives?

You can especially watch out for the theme of rebellion, which we described in the life story chapter (Doorway Two). Or are you someone who gets into trouble by always looking for rescuing to come from outside? Be aware of these themes. Then also be alert to contrary strands, perhaps not so prominent. If you have a prominent rebellion theme, look for the times when you also enjoyed being at ease with others and cooperating with them. See if you can find ways to encourage this cooperative aspect of yourself, as well as ways to express your rebellious self, that are not destructive. If you look for rescuing from outside, see if you can find times when you are acting out of the hero self.

PRACTICE

Identify the Chapters of Your Life

Here is another way to get in touch with the sweep of your life over time.

Sit and breathe consciously for a few moments with your journal open in front of you. Let your mind range over the sweep of your life, as though your life story were a novel. Then divide it into ten or twelve chapters. Give each a title. Write a sentence or so that summarizes your feelings about that period of time. Then quietly read over what you have written, breathing in and out. See if you can feel a sense of direction that provides any clues about how you came to be where you are now and where you might be going in the future.

This exercise can be done more than once. Try it again a few weeks or months from now. You will find that a different sense of the organization of your life emerges each time, depending on the background of your present mental state. If you are a little depressed, you might see your life in terms of losses and disappointments. When you are more happy, your successes and good fortune may be more prominent. Each set of chapter divisions provides a different angle and helps you to see your life from a multidimensional perspective, just as having the slightly different points of view of two eyes gives you depth perception.

Frogs Become Princes Every Day

In myths and legends, transformation occurs instantly. One wave of the magic wand, and the pumpkin becomes a royal carriage; one kiss from the princess, and the frog becomes a noble prince. The reason is that such stories come from the unconscious, and the unconscious is timeless. In real life, transformations are occurring all the time. Frogs are becoming princes every day. Only we do not recognize transformations as such because of the time factor. We are biased, counting as miracles only those things which occur instantaneously.

A journal can be a vehicle of transformation. You need only allow some time. Have some patience, and you can transform things you consider garbage into flowers. Have some patience, and you can become the Buddha that you in fact already are.

PRACTICE

Write Your Own Unique Life Line

This practice is another vehicle for identifying life themes. Sit before a piece of blank paper, and write down your earliest memory, going as far back into childhood as you can manage. There's a lot of variability regarding how early a memory people can recall. Some will remember things as early as two years of age, others not until they were ten or older. That's okay. Just start with what you can remember. Then record your age in years in the left margin next to that particular memory.

Then list all of the years of your life from that earliest memory up until age fifteen or sixteen, writing each number along the left margin of the page. For each year, fill in one thing that you remember from that age, one thing that stands out for you about that time. You do not need to write it out in full; just put it down telegraphically. For example, "that time the teacher scolded me in front of the class," or "the day I won the fifty-yard dash." If you have difficulty coming up with a memory from a specific age, remind yourself what was going on then. "Hmm, let's see. I was in fifth grade that year. That was the year we moved to Dayton . . . ," and so on. This will usually suffice to activate your memory network from that time.

When you are done, read over what you have written, taking your time. Look for memories that connect in some way. See if you can identify various themes: success/failure, strength/weakness, closeness/distance, rebellion/conformity, acceptance/rejection, and so on.

If you try this again at another time, you may get a different result, as with the life chapters practice, thus adding depth to your perspective.

Your journal is the friend that is always there. It is an outer representation of your own capacity for mindfulness and wisdom. It can be truly sacramental, "an outward and visible sign of an inward and spiritual grace."

Doorway Four

MEDITATING

As a hart longs for flowing streams,
so longs my soul for thee, O God.
My soul thirsts for God, for the living God.
                                    —Psalm 42

There's a center of quietness within, which has to be known
and held. If you lose that center, you are in tension and begin
to fall apart.
                    —Joseph Campbell, *The Power of Myth* (1988)

❧

Practice meditation to become more accepting of yourself and your
life. When you become more accepting of what hurts as well as more
aware of life's many positive aspects, you establish a firm spiritual
foundation for recovery.

❧

In my freshman year in college, I shared tight quarters with a
roommate who had very different habits. Pete tolerated my need
to meditate, but was more interested in hearing the Knicks game
on the radio. On one occasion, Pete returned in the middle of a medi-

tation period. When we discussed it later, he was surprised to learn that I had been aware of his returning. "What good is it then?" he asked—as if unawareness or obliviousness were the goal of meditation. Like many others, he imagined meditation to be a trancelike state where meditators lose complete awareness of the world around them.

Meditation is about slowing down and just being. Meditation is not a state of oblivion. It is about experiencing the moment in the here and now. It is a state of relaxed openness and awareness. It is being aware of what is going on—in your body, your feelings, your mind, your world. Periods of meditation will greatly enhance your daily mindfulness practice.

Meditation is the cornerstone of mindful living. At a retreat we attended in Santa Barbara, Thich Nhat Hanh was asked how long one should meditate. He responded, "All day." He was not implying that we sit on meditation cushions all day long. He meant that meditation, when carried into the daily activities in our lives, becomes mindfulness, and that mindfulness or mindful living is a form of meditation. Mindfulness is meditation away from the meditation seat; meditation is simply a period of mindfulness while one is free of other activity.

The Thirst for Wholeness

There is a longing in each of us, a place in the heart where we yearn for a perfection of peace. Some, like the psalmist, identify God as the object of that longing. Others, among them Buddhists, stalwartly prefer not to name it. They describe only the state of being at which they aim, calling it nirvana. But whether one names the nameless or refuses to name it, whether one even has a concept of the transcendent, all are propelled by the same inner restlessness, the same quest.

In less philosophical moods, we imagine that wealth or power, success or fame will give us happiness. And while these things are in themselves good—however maligned they may be for the destructive uses we make of them—they fail to bring the peace we seek. Instead of the simple harmony for which we yearn, life continually throws complexity and tension our way.

Addiction is a yearning for a lesser god, for something that provides a temporary cessation of the ache, but no real healing. Whether it is alcohol, drugs, food, sexuality, thrills, excitement, the ecstatic self-forgetfulness of falling in love, or any of a million other things, when this yearning attaches to lesser things, one becomes entangled in horrible, repetitious patterns—including the distinctive hell that is the essence of addiction. The thirst for wholeness, transcendence, peace, well-being, paradise, or nirvana cannot be quenched with alcohol or with any of these things. Whatever label you give it, this need must be met in some other way.

Part of the answer may indeed be that we need to come to an acceptance—even an appreciation—of the tension, disharmony, incompleteness, and imperfection of life. It is in these very things that the soul speaks to us most clearly, as Thomas Moore argues eloquently in *Care of the Soul* (1992). We need ways to be present with life as it is rather than as we prefer it to be, to appreciate what is here now rather than put life off into some imagined perfect future, or place it back into some idyllic past. But if we are to learn to dwell in the Eternal Present, we need a way to widen our hearts out to embrace difficulties, *a way to be fully and soulfully in our lives.*

One aspect of this is learning to embrace the very things we are tempted to discard. The divorce that left us bruised and battered, bitter and abandoned; the career crash that smashed us hard against some unpalatable realities; the imperfections and limitations of parents who failed to give us the perfect childhood to which we feel entitled—these very things are revelatory, cracking us open and forcing us to look deeper.

Yet one must honor the need for a deeper peace. One must honor the hunger and thirst to touch the Transcendent, to touch the Whole rather than the part. We require some way to center down and come to ourselves in our deepest and highest aspects, to see beyond what is visible with our normal, myopic, and fragmentary vision.

How can we keep our heads straight when the very ground we walk on shifts beneath us? For many, a key way to do that is meditation. Though meditation in particular has received increasing attention in recent decades, for many it still evokes images of some special religious calling—of monks wandering in hooded robes through medieval cloisters, or bearded, emaciated yogis sitting in perfect stillness and bliss. There is a sense that meditation is for special souls, not busy people struggling with the daily commute and raising families.

The notion that meditation and related practices is for special people is destructive.

You're Already Doing It

We have learned in our work with clients that the word *meditation* can be intimidating for some people. Sometimes when we suggest meditation, the initial reaction is something like, "Oh, I can't do *that!*" So instead, we just offer a "breathing exercise"—that is itself a form of meditation—and people feel more comfortable. So relax. Don't let yourself be intimidated by the word. If you have started doing the breath awareness practice we introduced in Doorway One, you are meditating already.

Quo Vadis?

One of the things I ask therapy clients is where they think their present struggles are leading them, what quality these struggles are calling forth from within them. Whether or not they have a good immediate answer to that, the question itself is important. The question suggests a teleological perspective on life problems. That is, it suggests that there is purpose in the painful symptoms we wish only to get rid of as quickly as possible.

Indeed, we can ask this question from a global perspective as well: What is the present world situation requiring of us? What is it asking us to learn? How is it asking us to grow or change perspective? One answer may be that these times require people who are centered and relaxed, and who can accomplish this without leaving the world to accomplish this centering. We do not so much need people to leave for mountain caves and monasteries as we desperately need people who can be present and mindful in the world, in *this* world, in *our* world. As Zen teacher Charlotte Joko Beck said in *Everyday Zen* (1989), the injunction to "chop wood, carry water" must become "make love, drive freeway."

We need earthy mystics. There will always be a place for special vocation, for people who are called to lives of solitude. In hidden ways these people hold the rest of us together more than we know. But when one considers the present time, that is not what we need most. We need monks and nuns of the world: men and women dedicated to peace, but who do ordinary activities like keeping a job, raising a family, helping with homework, and shopping for groceries.

Fortunately, you do not need to retire into prolonged or permanent solitude to find peace. Peace is available to us all, and can be integrated into everyday life. It really is possible. You can do it. You can learn to embody peace.

The speed and complexity of our lives continues to increase. There is no reason to believe this will change anytime soon. To counter it, we need to find a stillness within, and to find it right in the midst of our daily routine rather than in ways requiring dramatic change or relocation. Addiction and other forms of destructive behavior are symptoms of our increasingly stressful lives. Many find an antidote in meditation.

PRACTICE

Establish a Meditation Practice

The confusion of approaches to meditation can make it difficult to know how to begin. But whether you are considering establishing a meditation practice for the first time, wanting to reestablish a practice that has been lost, or have been meditating for many years, it is helpful to return to basics. After all, we are always learning to meditate. An attitude of openness and continual learning is best. Zen in fact teaches that learning is the proper state of mind to be in for sitting, that we are always beginning again. The mind of the enlightened person is exactly "beginner's mind"—open, soft, receptive, and available, not a full teacup.

Here is a basic set of instructions to start with (or return to):

1. Find a comfortable, quiet place.
2. Sit in a manner that allows you to be relaxed, but also alert. Sitting up straight avoids drowsiness and, according to many traditions, aligns centers of spiritual energy.

3. Let yourself settle in and center down. Take time. Start with being aware of what is around you, using all sense modalities: what you see, what you hear, smell, touch, and perhaps taste. Be aware of your feelings about what has been going on that day. Imagine your skin as that which *connects you to* everything, instead of that which separates you from it. Gradually tune more inward by focusing on your breathing, breathing gently in and out, experiencing each breath as a quiet and simple pleasure, making no effort to change or alter your breathing in any way, but just experiencing it.

4. Find a focal point for your attention. It can be concrete, such as the tip of a stick of burning incense or an image of a Buddha, a flower or a mountain; or it can be something you envision, such as the Inner Light of Quaker meditation. You can continue to just focus on the breath, as Zen teachers such as Thich Nhat Hanh instruct. You can use a word or phrase, either saying it out loud or repeating it silently to yourself. Or, as in Vipassana meditation, the focus can be the flow of your thoughts. The newer you are to meditation, or the more distracted you happen to be at a particular time, the more you may need something concrete to focus on.

5. Trust the process. Don't try to make anything special happen, or worry whether you are doing it right. Whatever happens is right for you, now. Be present with whatever happens. Meditation is nothing special—just a time to *be*.

6. Continue for a comfortable period of time. Ten minutes may be plenty if this is new to you. An hour may not feel like enough if you have been practicing for some time and have come to enjoy it.

There are, of course, endless variations in technique, but in our workshops we have found these procedures easiest for the majority of people.

How Meditation Helps

You may have heard of the *fight or flight response*. Our modern nervous system is not drastically different from that of early human beings. When a human being perceives a threat in the environment, the nervous system responds in ways well suited to the dangerous, wild savannas of our early human ancestors. Blood is shunted away from maintenance processes like digestion (giving us a knot in the stomach) in favor of the emergency needs of the large skeletal muscles. Blood pressure, respiration, and heart rate all increase. In essence, the body prepares to encounter danger, either by running away from it or fighting. This response served our ancestors well, allowing them to survive and pass these characteristics on to us.

The fight or flight response serves us well in few situations today. If you are camping in the mountains and encounter a hungry bear, it might be useful. However, it is detrimental in most other situations. If your boss is angry with you, the most effective response usually will not be to hit her, nor to run away. In fact, even with the bear, calmness may be more helpful, because running may trigger the aggressiveness you wish to prevent.

Driving is an everyday example of how the fight or flight response is not helpful. At rush hour, no matter how much you resolve to drive calmly and nonaggressively, it is difficult not to get caught up in the aggressiveness of other drivers. The frustration and anger of the road spread swiftly from car to car. When another driver does something unexpected, our nervous system responds in the same way as to the bear. Here, however, it is clearly not helpful. We can neither run away from this kind of threat nor fight. Though road rage is not the best thing for this situation, it is understandable in the sense that this it is exactly the "fight" part of fight or flight. It is in keeping with our physiology. Once this is triggered, we are then in the situation of struggling against our biological response patterns. To make it worse, while our central nervous system reacts quickly, the endocrine system—our glands and hormones—reacts less quickly and also shuts off less quickly. This means that the hormones involved in fight or flight, especially cortisol, epinephrine, and norepinephrine, pour into our bloodstreams. Even after we have reappraised the situation, and realize either that the danger is past, or that there was no real danger to begin with, these hormones remain active for some time, pushing us to fight or run, and leaving us exhausted when we can do neither. It is like psyching yourself up to get into the ring with Ali, only to find the fight has been canceled at the last minute. No wonder the daily commute is so tiring.

Meditation elicits a response opposite to the fight or flight response. Respiration and heart rate decrease. Blood pressure drops. Oxygen consumption plummets to ten or twenty percent below normal—lower in fact than in deep sleep. Harvard researcher Herbert Benson called this the *relaxation response* in his book of the same title (1975).

Think of it this way. The autonomic nervous system is that part of the nervous system over which we do not have direct, voluntary control. This part of the nervous system has two branches, sympathetic and parasympathetic. The sympathetic nervous system responds to threat, and mobilizes our defenses to run or fight. It is analogous to the gas pedal on your car. But your car would not be very useful if it only had a gas pedal and lacked a brake. Likewise, your body needs a brake to counter the gas pedal of the sympathetic nervous system. That brake is called the parasympathetic nervous system. It triggers the relaxation response, to slow things back down and repair the damage caused by the emergency gas pedal system.

To extend the analogy, if you continually rev your motor at high speed, it will not last long. The systems that protect against engine wear fail. Heat and friction grind down the moving parts. A motor continually subjected to such abuse will have a short life-span.

Yet for some of us, it is as if we are doing just this with our bodies and minds. We are constantly operating at high rev. If we lack other means, we may resort to alcohol or other drugs that calm this over-stressed system. We try to use these things as brakes. And indeed they work, in the short run. But they also introduce long-term problems that ultimately make the situation worse. What we really need to do is find the natural brakes that are already available.

Meditation is a natural brake. And unlike the trade-offs with drugs, there is no downside. Meditation is a natural state. It is just being—the simplest thing of all. Since we have spent so much of our time learning the opposite of just being, it requires a little persistence to unlearn these ingrained habits. But it is not hard to do, and the whole process of learning can be enjoyable. Benson found that novices at meditation, who had been practicing only for a few weeks or months, showed physiological changes almost as profound as those who had been meditating for fifteen or twenty years. So remember, *even if you are worrying that you might not be doing it right, your body and mind still benefit.*

Choose the Meditation Environment

While advanced meditators may be able to meditate virtually any-where, it is important to have a peaceful, quiet place, especially when learning. Turn off the phone, the radio, the television. Be away from others so there is no need to be self-conscious. Shut the door. There is little chance of having quiet inside without quiet outside.

Choose the place in your home for meditation practice carefully. To have a special place for meditation is helpful. This can be explained on different levels. On the level of the psychology of learning, there is conditioning. An environment associated with calmness and reduced tension elicits similar feelings when you return to it. On a spiritual level, you create a meditative atmosphere or energy in that place which helps you reenter meditative awareness. Whatever the explanation, it works.

At the same time, you will need to be able to take your meditation with you when you are away from home or when, for whatever reason, your accustomed place is unavailable. And even if you have a regular place for meditating, you might sometimes wish to meditate in special places—a church or temple, a place of historic spiritual interest like the site of the Buddha's enlightenment or the temple wall in Jerusalem—or a peaceful natural setting, such as a beautiful lake or mountaintop. Beverly and I find both special places and regular places helpful. Beverly particularly loves meditation in scenes of natural beauty, and I love my meditation spot at home. As always, experiment with what environments are most conducive, and discover your own optimal combination of regularity and novelty.

An Object of Meditation

As long as you or I are alive, we will be thinking. And as long as we are thinking, we will be thinking about something. There is no such thing as an inactive mind. Some describe meditation as a wave of thought about emptiness or nothingness, but even so, there is a wave of thought. The only question is whether the mind is focused or scattered, and *what* the mind is focused on.

One of the simplest ways to reach a meditative state is to focus on an object. The object can be anything: a flower, the glowing tip of a stick of incense, the image of a saint, one of the spiritual centers or chakras in the body, a spot on the floor. The "object" does not even need to be visual at all. An aroma, a sound, a sensation, or even, as we will discuss later, one's own thoughts. One of the easiest ways to start is with a sound, such as a word. But choose a word that appeals to you. Love, light, and peace are good candidates, because they evoke associations conducive to meditation. Some people love to use a prolonged *aaaahhh* or the Hindu holy word *Om*, drawn out sonorously and resonantly. Or try one of the ancient chants like *Om mane padme hum*. This means "the jewel is in the lotus," indicating the presence of enlightenment in the heart of all things, although for many it is not the meaning but the *sound* of this chant that is important. A little closer to home, try the Hebrew *Shema*: "*Shema Yisrael, Adonai Elohenu, Adonai Echad*" (Hear, O Israel: The Lord our God, the Lord is One), which may be seen as a profound statement of unity. The Hesychastic teaching of the Greek Orthodox Church focuses on the repetition of the prayer of Jesus, a short version of which goes, "Lord Jesus Christ, have mercy on me." Some Muslims repeat the name Allah over and over, increasing in volume and excitement to culminate in a state of ecstasy.

Benson's research demonstrated that the relaxation response is deeper when people tap into their own religious and spiritual beliefs. So choose a word or phrase or other object of attention that makes sense to you, that feels right, and for which you have positive associations—perhaps tapping your own religious heritage if it feels appropriate.

The most frequently used object of attention is the breath. When we focus on the breath, just allowing it to proceed of its own accord and not interfering, feeling each breath all the way in and all the way out, enjoying the way it refreshes and unifies body and mind, we tap physiological processes that are naturally calming and healing. The breath has the advantage of being always available to you, no matter where you are. It is possible with practice to learn to keep some attention on the breath and benefit from its calming effect even while doing other things. Whatever else you may use as an object of meditation, we suggest you consider working with conscious breathing as well.

PRACTICE

Experience the Breath as Happening of Itself

Some people get caught up in trying to control their breath in meditation and have difficulty just following it or experiencing it without interfering. To learn to let the breath just happen, you might enjoy this practice.

As you settle down and become aware of your breath, focus your attention a little more on the outbreath than on the inbreath. Notice that point of pause just after exhalation, and instead of *deciding* to breathe in, just let your body breathe in when it feels ready to—as deeply or as shallowly as it wants to. Experience the breath as just falling back into your body of its own accord, and then, at the inflection point after the inbreath, falling back out of its own accord.

Ask yourself, Am I breathing, or am I being breathed?

A Comfortable Position

Position is no trivial point. In Eastern traditions, a great deal of ingenuity has gone into finding optimal positions for meditation. The end result of that ingenuity is the full lotus position: seated with legs crossed and each foot resting on the opposite thigh. It is no accident that this position became popular. It is very stable, allowing one to sit very straight almost effortlessly. It is conducive to a state of meditation, because it is a posture that in itself expresses what we aim at in meditation: to be relaxed but effortlessly alert and aware. It is the opposite of lying down in that lying down is more conducive to sleep than to relaxed mindfulness.

The full lotus posture looks cool, you might think. It looks very impressive, very spiritual. It seems obvious that someone who can sit like that is much more advanced spiritually than someone who sits in a chair.

But forget appearances. Western backs and knees are generally not prepared for this posture. So it becomes self-defeating. Most Westerners who do manage to get into this position will be unable to think about much else besides how it hurts. And while being able to dwell with pain can be an important meditative practice, life brings enough opportunities to work on this without creating them artificially.

Naturally, if you can sit in the lotus or its modified version, the half lotus (legs crossed but only one foot resting on the opposite thigh), this is wonderful. If you can sit this way comfortably, it is without question the best posture for meditation. But it is the purpose of this posture that is essential. And the purpose of the lotus posture is to allow you to sit comfortably upright so that you can avoid drowsiness, while also being freed from strain or effort. If the posture itself is a strain or an effort, it does not serve its purpose. What you are really looking for is a way to sit comfortably, erect but not rigid. Find your own best way to do that, and you will have found what is essential.

Goals and Meditation Don't Mix

A passive attitude is the most important element of meditation. If meditation is approached like jumping jacks in high school physical education, it will not be pleasant. Furthermore, it will not be helpful. Avoid approaching meditation like eating that awful canned spinach our parents made us eat as children—because it is supposed to be good for us. Avoid a goal orientation, with dreams of nirvana dancing in your head, or an expectation of instantly solving all your dilemmas and problems. This is true of any means of fostering mindfulness we discuss in this book. But it especially applies here. If you must have goals, let them be simple: to feel a little more calm, to treat your body and mind to a few moments of quietness and relaxed attention. Not to become Gandhi—at least not in your first sitting.

Remember what we said about the nervous system itself. As described above, the relaxation response is a state of activation of the parasympathetic nervous system, the "brakes." Goal-oriented behavior is associated more with the voluntary nervous system and with sympathetic arousal. When you are making a sale to an important client, you perspire more, your heart beats faster, and you get a pit in your stomach—all signs of sympathetic nervous system activation. But this is not what you need in meditation. Goals and meditation don't mix.

The Best Way

What is the best way to meditate? We'll tell you a secret it took us a long time to learn. *The best way to meditate is to enjoy it.* Make it something you look forward to. You are treating yourself to a special time of relaxation and peace. Enjoy the quietness. If you hear of people who trek off to India for twenty years and meditate with some supreme guru with a secret, esoteric teaching, doing nothing but sitting for twenty-five hours a day and eating only one grain of rice, fine. If this is your path, let nothing divert you from it. But if you find that your meditation becomes a chore when you try to mediate for longer than ten minutes, then do your ten minutes and stop. Or better yet, do five minutes and stop. But let that five minutes be a totally restful, enjoyable experience. It is not how long you meditate, but how well. And how well you meditate depends upon being happy and enjoying the experience.

As soon as you introduce striving into your meditation, you are off the beam. If you are meditating one hour a day, and imagining just how incredible it would be if you meditated for two hours, slow down. Stick with your one hour until you can barely pull yourself away after that period of time. Concern about who is the most spiritual and who meditates the longest is of a piece with who drove the hottest car in high school. It simply does not fit with this activity. There are no levels. We are all Buddhas, and we are all learning. Striving is of the small self. Be gentle with the small self. Tell it you will take care of it in other ways. But keep it away from your meditation.

Opening the Heart

Thich Nhat Hanh tells of a woman who stubbornly persisted in her practice of invoking the name of the Buddha for an hour three times a day. She persisted in the practice for ten years. Her character, however, did not change. She was as mean as ever. To teach her a lesson, a friend

came to her door precisely when he knew she would be starting her
practice. As he called her name repeatedly, she fought with her irritation, trying to ignore him. Finally, she answered the door angrily,
demanding to know why her friend kept calling her name so many
times. The friend replied that if she was that angry after he called her
name, just think how angry the Buddha must be after ten years!

Someone asked the aging Aldous Huxley what the effect of his
years of study of Eastern religion and his practice of meditation was.
He replied that perhaps it had made him a little kinder. Similarly, the
Tibetan tradition is full of secret, esoteric teachings. Yet when the
Dalai Lama describes the essence of his own religion, he insists that
his religion is kindness.

The purpose of a meditation practice is to make us less hard, less
brittle, more in rhythm with the Tao—the underlying harmony of the
cosmos. It is for opening the heart. It is practicing nonviolence toward
ourselves, our thoughts and feelings, and the world around us. If we
approach meditation practice in a hard or rigid way, if we approach it in
a driven way, with competitiveness and with an achievement attitude, it
is just more of the same, and not the healing enterprise we need.

The best way to approach meditation is with delight, with enjoyment, and with a gentle, Buddha-like smile. Sit in meditation just to
enjoy sitting. Make the most progress by seeking no progress whatsoever.

The Meditative Atmosphere

It can help your meditation if you create a conducive atmosphere
around you. One of the things that can help, as discussed above, is
constancy of place. Meditating in the same place regularly, if possible,
helps trigger the relaxation response. Constancy of time can also be
helpful. Doing your meditation at the same time of day each day
establishes a helpful rhythm.

Many report that the best times for meditation are morning and
evening. There is a story that the famed Indian sitar player Ravi
Shankar commented on a concert he was to give in the afternoon. He
could hardly fathom playing at such a nonspiritual time. And while we
feel that you can meditate anytime, it does seem the case that morning
and evening are especially conducive. Meditation in the morning can

establish a mood and intention for the day ahead. Meditation in the evening can help you process the day's events and the associated stress and leave it behind. As always, experiment and see for yourself. And of course, meditating in the afternoon is better than not meditating, if that is the only alternative.

It also helps to have objects that establish the right mood around you when you meditate. Choose things that evoke a feeling of sacredness and peace. Perhaps an icon of a saint, a painting of the Christ, or a blissful and happy-looking Buddha. Perhaps objects that do not have specifically religious connotations but that help you feel peaceful and centered.

Burning incense is another aid in meditation. Smell is a primitive sense connected with deep, older parts of the human brain. It is also a connection with ancient rituals that originally involved animal sacrifice. One of the marks of deep, authentic mystical experience is smell, as many recorded mystical experiences testify. The "scent of holiness" is more than a phrase. Scent grabs us at a profound level. The use of incense in many traditions is not accidental. And again, on the level of psychological conditioning, if you meditate with a certain scent around you, then that scent can trigger the meditative state more easily in the future.

Sound is another sensory dimension that can help. We have already discussed chanting or repeating words or phrases. Some people find it useful to have peaceful, quiet music in the background, or to use a tape of guided meditation. We have a tape of people chanting *Om* that we like, especially if it helps block out other sounds that might be distracting. Best of all, perhaps, is the "sound of silence"—that almost palpable silence that you can find in quiet, natural settings. But if you live on a busy street, a soothing tape may be better than the background noise. Here as always, do what really works for you, and do not be bothered by whether it conforms to some image of what you think is supposed to be best or most spiritual.

In our home, we have a simple altar as our meditation center. On the altar are some special objects, "props" that are meaningful to us and conducive to a meditative atmosphere. There is a bell, an incense holder, a sage stick, a little statue of a peaceful Buddha sitting in meditation, a statue of Saint Francis, a couple of crystals. We have cushions for when we want to sit on the floor, and a sofa we sit on when that feels better. Over time, objects are added or removed as we find other things we like, that evoke the right kind of feelings in us. This altar provides a focal point in our home. We can and do sometimes meditate in other places, but this particular place is the center, the heart of our home. If you do not have such a center where you live, you might like to create one.

Catherine de Hueck Doherty, writing out of the Russian Orthodox tradition, talks about *poustinia*, a Russian word for desert and the title of her book (1975). In this book she discusses the deep human need for desert, for places of solitude and silence and prayer. The Judeo-Christian spiritual traditions are full of imagery of the desert or wilderness, places where human beings are not, where one confronts, and is confronted by, oneself and God. In the Hindu religion, it is the forest. In Tibetan Buddhism, it is remote mountain caves, splendid in their solitude.

Poustinia does not need to be a literal desert. *Poustinia* in the Western world is also available in places you might not otherwise recognize as such: the *poustinia* of the commute to work, of standing in line at the supermarket, of waiting in the anonymity of the motor vehicle office. *Poustinia* is also the place you appoint as the place of silence and solitude and peace, that room or corner of a room that becomes part of you. *Poustinia* is that place in your heart, the inner sanctuary, the Shekinah of the soul. Such a place is all but essential for meditation or prayer.

A few minutes of quiet reading also helps make the transition to a meditative mood. Collect whatever books seem helpful to you for this purpose. Devotional classics or works about meditation are obvious choices, but it is not the subject matter so much as it is how it affects you. Be alert for surprises. If you love cooking, and reading cookbooks happens to get you into a very peaceful frame of mind, then cookbooks may be part of your meditation library.

There is always the danger with reading, however, that you can end up reading too long and substituting it for meditating. Accept no substitute. Be careful not to let reading and other preliminaries take up too much time from the thing itself. Just do it.

If we had to limit our advice to one word, that word would be *simplicity*. Keep it simple. There are endless numbers of mantras to chant, words to dwell on, techniques for visualization for centering. At one point, I found that I had accumulated so many techniques for centering down into my meditation that my whole meditation period was taken up with preliminaries.

Watch out for anything that introduces an element of strain. If your practice is to chant for twenty minutes, but you find yourself reluctant to do so and really having to push through it, try chanting inwardly and silently. If the process becomes too vague and unfocused, you can return to your chanting out loud briefly to give it greater solidity, then go back to silent chanting. Or try something else altogether, such as visualizing the Inner Light at the level of the heart chakra. Be pragmatic. Techniques are just techniques. There is nothing sacrosanct about any one approach. What matters is what gets you to that place of peaceful attention.

Dealing with Distractions

Okay, so you're ready to meditate. You sit down, collect yourself, and begin to focus on your word or other focal point. But your mind drifts off into a fog. Or you keep replaying an upsetting incident at work. In any case, you do not feel you are where you want to be for your meditation session.

Through the ages, many wise people have dealt with this problem. The anonymous fourteenth-century author of *The Cloud of Unknowing* wrote that when it becomes difficult to meditate, one should resort to whatever special tricks or techniques are helpful. "It is best," he wrote, "to learn these methods from God by your own experience rather than from any man in this life." There is that within you that will help you find your way, and you may discover helpful things unique for your temperament and situation. Be open to inventing useful approaches yourself. The Christ, the Buddha, the Master Teacher is available to you at all times.

Nonetheless, the author of the *Cloud* shares some tips about this problem. His advice about distractions is to cover them "with a thick cloud of forgetting, as if they never existed," and to continue to do this if the thoughts continue. An alternative he recommends is to say *no* to them when distracting thoughts arise. Intriguingly, here he anticipates by more than six hundred years a technique in modern cognitive psychology called thought stopping, in which you imagine yourself shouting *no* at unwanted negative thoughts. You may not want to picture yourself shouting exactly, since this is a little violent for meditation. But a gentle "no" or "not now" may help. Or remind yourself: "I can deal with this later if I want to."

When you employ such techniques, however, you are in a situation fraught with paradox. Meditation is a process that unfolds naturally. When you evaluate whether you are doing it right, and perhaps decide you aren't, and then try to do something to control the process and get back on track, you create division. Now you have a struggle within yourself—a struggle between your desire to meditate in a certain way, and the reality of what is actually occurring. For this reason, if you use a technique to get your wandering, monkey mind back on track, this needs to be done with gentleness and patience. Struggle and strain are inimical to meditation.

Vipassana meditation—sometimes called insight meditation—unties this paradoxical knot in an intriguing way. In this type of meditation, the focus is on the stream of thoughts that pass through your mind. You can get a feel for this type of meditation if you sit for a few minutes and label your thoughts. For example: "Okay, I'm sitting here, and I'm going to label my thoughts. . . . I'm wondering if my friend is going to call me about lunch. Now I am worrying about what is right to do in this situation, whether to cancel because of the icy roads. Now I am wondering why they don't do more road clearing here in New Mexico. There is a feeling of anger or irritation about this. . . ." The idea is to be with each thought and feeling as it arises, letting each come and then letting it go, not clinging to any particular thought or feeling that might be called pleasant, nor avoiding any thought or feeling that is unpleasant.

This approach performs a kind of judo on the problem of distractions. Whereas in judo, you use the force generated by your opponent for your own purposes, so here you use the very force of these wandering thoughts against themselves. Eventually, they calm down. However, that should not really even be said, because to say that thoughts calm down introduces a goal and leads back to the same knots. All that needs to be said is, stay with the thoughts themselves. Follow them with quiet, gentle attention. Don't try to hold on to pleasant thoughts, and don't avoid unpleasant ones. Let them come and go.

Downshifting

Eventually, a shift begins to occur. But it occurs through not seeking any kind of shift, through accepting whatever the mind conjures up. The shift may be described as a figure-ground shift. Perhaps you have seen drawings such as those in introductory psychology texts which illustrate this principle. In one famous example, you see either a vase, or two human faces in silhouette, depending on which part of the painting you are seeing as foreground and which part you are seeing as background. For some people, it is hard to make the shift. But once you get it, you can begin to move back and forth between the alternate perspectives.

One way to describe what happens in insight meditation is that such a shift emerges spontaneously. By gently and patiently following your thoughts, another perspective becomes activated. Instead of seeing your thoughts as foreground, something else that is normally background comes into the foreground. This "something else" has been called Mind, or the Ground Luminosity. You could call it God in Paul Tillich's sense of God as the Ground of Our Being. Zen teachers prefer not to talk about it much, since by talking about it you introduce a goal and thereby a state of conflict and tension, and endless, confounding paradoxes.

Of course, if you get tied up in knots about this intriguing paradox, you probably can imagine what the instruction is: Follow these very thoughts, the ones about the knots themselves.

In practice, following thoughts is not always easy. Some take to this approach more readily than others do. As with all approaches, experiment. Be pragmatic. See if it is helpful to you. This approach may not be helpful for people who are depressed, or who have obsessive tendencies (a pattern of intrusive, unwanted thoughts). The person with depressive tendencies is already too focused on depressive thinking. Focusing on this even more could be helpful in the long, long run, but might increase the depression in the meantime. And by

definition, a person with obsessional tendencies gets tied up in difficult thought knots. Quite possibly, this approach could intensify that
problem. There need be no fear in trying it, however.

PRACTICE

Learn Not to Struggle

Sit in a place and manner conducive to meditation. Breathe
consciously for a few minutes, letting your awareness settle a
bit, like a flat stone settling slowly toward the cool bottom of a
deep lake. Then practice just noticing what is going on in your
mind and body. Label each thing you notice, and add the
phrase "and that's okay." For example:

> "Worrying about money . . . and that's okay."
> "Song from the radio still playing in my head . . . and
>   that's okay."
> "Tightness in my neck and shoulders . . . and that's
>   okay."
> "Car racing by outside . . . and that's okay."
> "Feeling sad . . . and that's okay."
> "Feeling calm . . . and that's okay."

Use this practice whenever you find yourself struggling
with distraction. Be sure you are not just saying "and that's
okay" mechanically, but use the words to practice letting it
really be okay.

Walking Meditation

Walking meditation can be delightful. It also is a natural bridge
between the passivity of sitting and the activity of our daily life. If we
can bring a meditative awareness to walking, it may help us learn to do
other things in a meditative way.

To begin walking meditation, pause in a standing position before
starting. Take a few conscious breaths, collecting yourself. Let your

awareness fall into the soles of your feet. Take a breath, and then as you breathe out, take a slow, natural step. Feel your foot caressing the earth as it makes contact. Then, when you are ready to breathe in, make a step with your other foot. Simply enjoy the act of walking, and the contact between your foot and the earth. Try not to take your worries for a walk with you.

If you are walking outside, you might like to walk a little bit faster so as not to call attention to yourself. You will need to take more steps with each inbreath and outbreath, but you can still do this mindfully. If you see something you enjoy, such as a beautiful tree, a flower, or children playing, you might like to pause to enjoy it for a while before returning to your walking.

Metta Meditation

All the great spiritual traditions teach the importance of love. But saying that it is a good practice to love is often easier than doing it. Metta meditation is a way of training yourself to become more capable of loving. Being a loving person utterly transforms your outer and inner life.

In metta meditation, it is important to practice love toward ourselves first of all. Only if we love ourselves will we have the capacity to love anyone else. What is more, since we are all far more connected than we imagine, loving ourselves is ultimately not a different thing from loving others.

When you practice metta meditation, breathe in and out and silently state some kindly intentions toward yourself as you do so. For example:

> May I be happy and joyful.
> May I have all I want and need.
> May I have ease of well-being.
> May I be free from harm or injury.
> May I be free from fear, worry, sadness, and all afflictions.
> May I attain peace (enlightenment).

Take your time. Continue to breathe in and out until you feel the effect of this and are able to feel loving toward yourself. When you can do this, you can then expand your meditation to the person you love most in the world, such as your partner, or to those you feel closest to, such as your family. Use the same words as above and simply substitute the name of the person who is the object of your metta meditation for the word *I*.

When you are ready, you can then sequentially move on to friends, then a neutral person, then someone you have difficulty with, and finally to all beings, taking your time at each level. Each level is a little harder than the one before it, and depends on the depth you reach at the previous level, so do not rush it. You do not have to try to get through all the levels at once.

It is especially nice to do metta meditation before you go to bed. When you feel loving and connected to the world in this way, you sleep easier.

Urge Surfing: Nancy's Story

Just as fighting off distracting or unwanted thoughts in meditation can introduce a sense of struggle and tension that is not helpful, so also tension and struggle are introduced by fighting off an urge to indulge in addictive or other unwanted behaviors.

Consider Nancy. Nancy has a drinking problem. She is on her way to shop for clothes at the mall when she passes a bar where she used to drink. Being in places associated with drinking often sets off urges, whether just a minor itch, or a powerful and all but irresistible impulse. Obviously, this is a danger point—a "slippery place" where she could easily fall.

The usual practice is to try to squelch the urge directly. Nancy could do this by pushing it out of awareness and attending to something else instead. Perhaps, for example, she could turn up the radio and sing along with it, using that as a distraction to keep her mind off drinking. Or she could focus on the shopping she is going to do.

Sometimes distraction is useful to at least get us through a tight situation. The problem is that often things that we try to reject have a way of returning with greater power. It is like being told not to think of elephants because even a brief thought about elephants will lead to drastic consequences. What happens? Immediately pachyderms prance through your awareness. If you had a thought about elephants without this fear attached to it, the thought could come and go. But the very fact that one has introduced an instruction *not* to think about elephants creates fear and attachment to these thoughts. In this way, the thoughts about elephants gain power. As a general rule, *that which is denied gains power.*

This is one of the difficult aspects of trying to change behaviors that have an addictive aspect. The more we struggle against them directly, the more power they gain. It is like being caught in a net: the more you struggle to free yourself, the more entangled you become. In fact, that is one reason we focus in this book on a healing way of life more than on addiction per se. Fighting the addiction directly can increase its power.

What, then, is the way out? One answer has to do with the Vipassana technique of following thoughts, without clinging or aversion. See the urge as just another thought, like other thoughts. It has no more reality or substance than other thoughts do. It is simply old karma, old conditioning. It is possible to be with an urge without the fear, to watch this thought come and to watch it go, neither nourishing it nor rejecting it. To do this even one time with an urge is a significant step, a real loosening of the grip of habit. When one adopts this attitude, when the fear is removed, relapse thoughts lose power.

Nancy's inner dialogue went like this. "Hmm . . . there's Sculley's. Boy, it sure was fun to hang out there. I wonder how everyone is doing? Wish I could stop in for a drink. Oh no! I don't want to do that! . . . Or do I? Would it really be so bad to just have one drink? What do I want to do with this? Maybe I could practice being with these thoughts, paying attention to them. I notice a feeling of tension. It's in my back and shoulders. Look, my mouth is salivating, imagining the taste of the beer. There's a feeling of fear. Interesting . . . a very powerful urge. Reminding myself to breathe gently in and out . . . Notice the thoughts, the feelings, the sensations. It seems to be diminishing now, slowly. I'm having a thought of impatience, wishing it would stop now. That's okay, I'll be with that, too. Now I'm having the thought that I can be with these feelings and not have to indulge them. It's okay to feel this and I can still choose not to drink. It's hard! But it's losing strength now. Breathing . . . Having thoughts now about the clothes I want to buy, and which store I should try first . . . More thoughts about Sculley's, but much less strong. Having a thought that

I'm past it now anyway and don't want to turn around. A feeling of freedom now . . ."

This approach, called "urge surfing," is a way of doing judo on urges. It directly parallels what thought following does with distracting thoughts in meditation. The enemy has been embraced, and is, because of this, no longer an enemy. If you are not driving, you can sit and close your eyes and breathe gently in and out, and allow these thoughts to be, watching them as they slowly lose power. Most of the time, the first twenty minutes of an urge is the really hard part. By "surfing" the urge, riding out the wave and going with its energy rather than trying to oppose it, you can avoid giving more power to such thoughts. It is easier to do this, however, if you have practiced with other kinds of thoughts prior to using it to deal with urges, when it is part of an overall approach to life of gentle mindfulness and peace.

Prayer

Prayer is simply *coming into the Presence*, whether you think of that Presence as Brahman, the Inner Light, or the Lord of Hosts. What is vital is being in that sacred space in which you know yourself to be in contact with the Transcendent. In keeping with this, a Jewish mystical tradition refers to God as "The Place."

One way to bring your meditation into harmony with your own religious beliefs is to use phrases from your own tradition as the focus of your meditation. Alternatively, your meditation practice may best be thought of as simply being in the Presence. Simplicity itself.

Trust the movements of the soul. If you find yourself praising God or asking for God's help with some problem and talking it out, let it happen. Let it happen, even if this does not fit your philosophy. If you do not believe in God or believe only in a very abstract kind of God, but in some movement of the soul find yourself on your knees crying "Father" or "Mother," stand aside and let it happen. Or if you believe in a very personal God, but find your attention riveted on some impersonal aspect, let it happen. Trust the experiencing more than your philosophy. As noted psychologist Carl Rogers wrote, "Neither the Bible nor the prophets—neither Freud nor research—neither the revelations of God nor man—can take precedence over my own direct experience." Or as one Zen master put it: "Put no head above your own." That would include not putting your own ideas of what you should experience above what you actually do experience.

Keep It Simple

This book presents a spiritual path based on wholeness and healing through mindfulness. To find the way out of addictive behaviors and other problems, it helps to become more deeply aware. With deeper awareness, you see options where none existed before. Doors open out of stone walls.

Meditation can help. While we can only sketch some of the basics in this brief chapter, you do not need a lot of knowledge to begin. Begin where you are, with the information at hand. If you desire to learn more, there are plenty of excellent manuals about meditation. Nearly every community has meditation centers these days. Help and support are not hard to find.

We are not inclined to say that any practice is absolutely necessary or indispensable. However, we stop just short of doing that in the case of meditation. If there is an essential practice, meditation is it.

Whatever you do, refuse to encumber the process of meditation with a heavy overlay of technique or with requirements that feel burdensome. Do not allow your time of meditation to become a heavy "should," another "have to." Follow your Inner Teacher. Keep your practice joyful, and keep it simple. Learn to appreciate the wisdom of passivity and receptivity.

Allow.

Let.

Relax.

Trust.

Be.

Doorway Five
RECREATION AND NATURE

Ten thousand flowers in spring, the moon in autumn,
a cool breeze in summer, snow in winter.
If your mind isn't clouded by unnecessary things,
this is the best season of your life.
          —Wu-men, *Wu-men-Kuan*, 1228

∞○∞

Find ways to connect with the natural world. Addicted people are often alienated from the natural world. A return to nature is incompatible with addiction. Conscious, mindful choices about your recreational time prevent you from squandering it on passive pursuits that do not employ your higher human qualities, such as intellectual, artistic, and spiritual activities.

∞○∞

By late afternoon, Catherine has already begun thinking about her first glass of wine after work. To her coworkers, she seems quite normal; they hardly suspect she's just going through the motions. She attends to her secretarial tasks in a superficial, unconscious fashion. But behind her expressionless mask, she is simply wishing time away, watching the hour hand move ever so slowly toward five.

Jimmy survives the workweek by living for the weekend. His is a fantasy world full of exciting, recreational daydreams. The workweek is simply the unfortunate bridge between weekends—a kind of mandatory filler that he has grown accustomed to and accepts as an annoying fact of life. Just as a child sees brussels sprouts as an unavoidable nastiness between meat and dessert, Jimmy sees work as an interruption to his real life.

The weekend for Jimmy is a time for parties, watching sports on television, and generally letting go. He is seeking to replicate the grand old time he had in college. His Saturday nights never quite live up to his expectations, so what does he do? He tries harder. Jimmy restlessly seeks the exciting level of fun seen in sitcoms and action movies, but so glaringly absent in real life.

He consistently finds that he overindulges on weekends and eats and drinks too much, but somehow this has also become one of the necessary ingredients for the weekend. These weekends rarely meet his expectations, but Jimmy continues in pursuit of his mythic good time. Not only does this myth somehow never quite fulfill itself, but it has terrible costs. Jimmy misses five days out of every seven of his life. And Sundays are full of anticipatory dread and depression as he contemplates returning to work Monday morning.

Work and Play

Recovery is so much more than abstinence. Quitting is an important and difficult first step. But however important it is, it is not enough. We cannot overemphasize that successful recovery ultimately requires a more balanced, harmonious lifestyle rather than just a direct attack on the drugs or alcohol.

Mindful living is simply incompatible with excessive consumption or bingeing. The more mindful each of us becomes, the less we indulge in excess. The more mindful we become, the more we see that even when we do slip and indulge ourselves, we are not in the expected throes of blissful enjoyment. We become increasingly aware that bingeing doesn't feel good. When we become more aware, it is not the pleasure we imagine it to be. At the same time, we learn to pay more attention to simple, natural, everyday pleasures. We develop the capacity to live every moment of every day instead of just weekends and vacations.

If we try to simply "pull ourselves up by our bootstraps," forcing abstinence while maintaining the same unsatisfying lifestyle, we are bound to fail. If we spend our weekdays at joyless work, we create an imbalance. This imbalance creates a pressure to make the nonwork time special and rewarding, including a craving for distraction—distraction from unfulfilling and meaningless jobs. At the end of a day of empty work, there's a sense that we have to make up for it somehow, that we have to fill ourselves to compensate for the drudgery.

It is not enough to just live for the weekends. Life is precious. Every moment deserves our full attention. Every moment deserves to be lived deeply and fully. Unsatisfying work leads to unsatisfying recreation. We need to break the cycle.

In *The Revinvention of Work* (1994), Matthew Fox describes the alienation we experience when we let ourselves get stuck in unsatifying work:

> It is time we take back our entertainment hours from the captains of the entertainment industry. Think about how much of our leisure time we surrender to professional athletes and their corporate sponsors rather than to our own needs for exercise and relaxation. . . . We need to take up activities that truly engage us with ourselves and others—music, painting, poetry, dance, massage, cooking, hiking in nature—not to pursue prizes or with a mentality of judgment but rather as we would approach prayer itself, for that is what these actions are: acts of meditation and art as meditation.

The deep split between work and the rest of life must be healed. It is not enough to try to compensate for the living death of meaningless work with equally empty entertainment. Our time at work is also life. It needs redemption from emptiness. But equally in need of redemption is the time wasted in what passes for amusement and entertainment.

Recreation is not synonymous with distraction. Satisfying leisure time rarely comes from wild parties and outrageous movies. Leisure time that makes us feel good is more commonly full of simple pleasures. When you learn to contemplate a flower with full awareness, you are more happy than you can imagine. You touch more happiness through such simple acts than is possible through any prepackaged entertainment.

Have you ever invited friends over for dinner and for no apparent reason experienced a superbly perfect evening? Many years ago, Beverly entertained old friends for dinner. After a full day of chasing a toddler, she was too exhausted to lavishly entertain. She put together a simple stew, and barely straightened the house before company arrived. But the evening felt perfect, because the time was spent with good friends engaged in meaningful conversation. Elaborate meals served in immaculate homes do not guarantee a joyful evening and sometimes even get in the way by shifting the focus onto superficial concerns.

Separation from the Natural World

Who are we? What is our true nature? The Zen koan asks, What did our face look like before our parents were born? We are not just the roles we play at work with our coworkers, or the masks we wear at home with partners and family. We are not those creatures propelling themselves across town in their automobiles. We are part of it all; we are the all. We are part of nature, and we are nature.

PRACTICE

See Yourself and the World as Not Two

Sit in meditation posture and breathe in and out a few times, resting comfortably and enjoyably in the breath. Then, instead of seeing yourself as a separate part of the world, isolated and alone, imagine for a while that your skin *connects* you to the rest of the world around you instead of separating you from it. With your eyes closed, still breathing in and out, sense the world around you, beginning with your immediate surroundings. Feel yourself as connected, not really separate at all from these surroundings. Gradually let this sense of unity or not-twoness extend to the whole earth, then to the whole universe.

When you are ready to conclude this practice, point your finger at your own chest and say to yourself, "Now I am going to point at myself." Let this intention become firm and clear.

Then, as you open your eyes, point away from yourself. During the rest of the day, see if you can hold on to some of this sense of connectedness.

The present degree of separation between human beings and the natural world is unprecedented. We have come so far, achieved such miracles, but have sacrificed so much along the way. We have given up the essential connection to the great outdoors. We have lost the vital sense of unity and interdependence with nature.

Most of us in today's society do not till the soil and plant crops in order to earn our way in the world. But we cannot exist without the natural world. The very cells in our body scream when another acre of rain forest is cleared. And this is not mere metaphor. The chemical structure of the hemoglobin in our blood that carries oxygen to our cells is exactly the same as the chlorophyll in plants, the chemical that converts sunlight into plant energy, except for one single central molecule. The chemical that feeds the plants is virtually the same thing as the chemical that feeds our cells.

As a young girl growing up in Boston, Beverly thought milk, cheese, and beef came directly from the supermarket wrapped in cellophane. She could not connect these items with cows and farms, so foreign to her experience. As adults, we know this is not so, and we can find such a childish perception amusing. But it is not so amusing; it betrays how far removed from the natural life process we all have become.

Mother Earth

A hundred years ago, most people farmed or otherwise lived off the land. They did not need to manufacture exercise programs to stay in shape or to expend calories. They got their daily aerobic activity from their work. They walked, lugged supplies, mended fences, washed clothes by hand, and were physically active most of the day. Just imagine the absurdity of farmers in the early 1900s getting up and jogging for an hour in the morning, or working out with weights three times per week. They had no need to artificially create exercise programs. The farmer's job and way of life were one; his work was one big, natural exercise program.

Most human beings a hundred years ago did not have to invent ways of spending time outdoors in nature. In addition to providing them with ample exercise, their daily labor placed them outdoors in nature much of the time. They earned a living from the land and had continuous contact with Mother Earth. Every day they experienced the true source of the things we find in the supermarket.

We are renewed by contact with the soil. The mythological giant Antaeus challenged men to wrestle with him in a life-or-death struggle. He drew the strength for victory by simply touching Mother Earth. He was renewed by contact with the soil. Knowing the source of Antaeus's strength, Hercules could only defeat him by holding him in the air, choking him, and refusing him the life-sustaining contact with the earth.

With Herculean power, modern life keeps us removed from the earth. We let our vitality be choked out of us. Our jobs, our automobiles, our computers, all conspire to diminish time spent in nature. Or perhaps more accurately, we permit our careers and our electronic toys to take precedence over our time spent outdoors.

Our computers and automobiles, our televisions and modern appliances, are not bad in and of themselves. We can barely imagine modern life without them. They have become virtual necessities. But our electronic, computerized lives present us with a mountain of manufactured obstacles that we must climb in order to reconnect with nature. Since a restoring, revitalizing contact with nature no longer just happens during the course of our daily lives, communing with nature requires a conscious and deliberate choice.

PRACTICE

Use Television Mindfully

Probably the main source of passive entertainment for most of us is television. We are attracted to its warm, comforting glow. It seems to make no demands of us. It bombards us with disturbing images, and feeds cravings of all kinds through flashy advertising sounds and sights.

For a period of time, a day, a week, or a month—whatever feels comfortable—give special attention to taking control of your television viewing. Use the television listings as a tool of mindfulness, and decide ahead what you really want to watch. Then turn it off when that particular program is over.

Notice what happens as a result of this experiment. How do you use the time? Do you end up talking more with family members? Do you read more, or listen to music? Do you go for a stroll in the evening? Practice mindful breathing? How does this feel in comparison with the way you normally use television?

What We Take for Granted

Beverly worked with mentally ill prison inmates who, of course, are denied many freedoms. But of all the things they miss, you might not guess what they miss the most. Although many of these inmates have a history of alcohol and substance abuse, most do not report that alcohol or their drug of choice is what they long for. They do not pine for a cold beer, a scotch on the rocks, or a line of cocaine. *They miss the freedom of being outdoors in nature.* They miss taking a walk in the woods. They miss hiking in the mountains. They miss camping, fishing, and swimming. In short, they miss all of the beauty of the natural world that they took for granted most of their lives. Because we have the feeling that these things are there whenever we want, we pay little attention to them.

Ralph Waldo Emerson put it succinctly when in 1849 he wrote:

If the stars should appear one night in a thousand years, how would men believe and adore; and preserve for generations the remembrance of the city of God which had been shown!

However, stars do not shine once in a thousand years, but instead provide us with a nightly spectacle. So how do we appreciate this grand display? Do we daily profess awe and gratitude for it? Are we overcome with the majesty of these distant, scintillating suns? No. Generally we forget to look up. Like the friend who is always there, we take the stars for granted and seldom appreciate their beauty.

Unless we cultivate mindfulness, it is all too easy to lose awareness of the miracles right in front of us. In order to function effectively in this world, we often become inured to its ugliness—the squalor of inner-city poverty, the murders and rapes on the nightly news, the dilapidated city buildings, the trash on the sidewalk. But when we mute our sensibilities enough to tune out the negative aspects, we also lose our appreciation for the beautiful.

The human nervous system has a built-in tendency to get used to things that are frequently present. We barely notice the sound of the clock ticking, the rushing air of our cooling or heating systems, or the background hum of fluorescent lights. Psychologists call this phenomenon *habituation*. To some extent, it serves a useful purpose. When you are able to shut out the ticking clock, you are free to notice other things.

Unfortunately, however, we habituate most easily to the positive elements of our experience. Things that go wrong never fail to capture our attention, but we hardly notice the countless things that go right every day. At a beautiful, clear mountain lake, the single rusted beer can along the shore grabs our attention more than the play of light and wind on the water or the wildflowers blooming outrageously at water's edge.

Meditating to notice the flowers is not just poetry. Some research has shown that experienced Zen-style meditators, who practice becoming deeply aware of the present moment, do not habituate to repetitive stimuli. Each time the clock ticks, it is heard fresh and new. Meditation teaches us to see the flowers and stars as though we had never seen them before and would never see them again.

Celebrate Life

So if it were all taken away from us as in some science fiction fantasy, how would we react and what would we care about? If we were threatened with the end of the world, with mass destruction of the earth by the devastation of war or by monstrous villains, we would cry out against the annihilation of our beautiful world. When faced with losing this beauty we take for granted, we would rise up at the horror of never again seeing the trees, a beautiful sunset, or the magnificent ocean.

Once a taxi driver told Beverly that some months earlier, he had suddenly become seriously ill and for a brief time was paralyzed from the neck down. The doctors were not sure what was causing the paralysis and told him that they could not predict whether it would be permanent. He faced the prospect of never being able to walk, exercise, throw a ball in the park, drive a car, or even move at all.

The paralysis, however, disappeared as quickly as it had come, and he was gratefully well again. He now knew the fleeting, impermanent, precious nature of life. He knew to appreciate the wonders of the natural world. For the ability to enjoy nature and to play in the great outdoors can be snatched away in an instant.

When he was released from the hospital, he told his family that it was time to travel. He would not continue to postpone that long awaited cross-country trip. They would celebrate life by visiting the scenic wonders this country has to offer. Gone were the excuses for not making this dream a reality. He would no longer dismiss his desires as folly, and would savor the life he almost lost.

Please do not wait until your body fails you to enjoy the natural world.

We Are Part of Nature

One day while I was meditating with eyes closed, feeling particularly relaxed, I felt a presence. Opening my eyes partway, I saw one of our neighborhood cat friends making his rounds down the sidewalk before our front windows. The grace and ease of his movements brought a smile to my whole body. I also noticed the plants in our living room, and for a few moments, I knew that I was one with plants, cat, and whatever else was around and in my awareness. The cat was not experienced as something that might use our garden again for its litter box, and the plants were not just there as something that might need watering and tending. They, and I, existed for ourselves. In a moment of deep meditative calm, there was an opening to this new level of reality. It was almost as though everything shimmered with light.

This type of experience is nothing unique. It is available to all of us, because we do not exist apart from our natural environment. As human beings, priding ourselves on being advanced members of the animal kingdom, we are still part of nature. The existence of one thing implies the existence of the whole universe. When you eat an apple, you contact the sunshine and soil and water, the roots and leaves, the workers who made the apple available to you, and all the elements that nourished the apple. When you eat an apple, you touch the universe. You are God taking God into God.

Plants provide us with life-sustaining oxygen and beautify our world. We require water and sunlight for survival and use natural resources such as trees and earth to construct houses for shelter. We cannot live without the earth and its many gifts. Repressing our connection to the environment creates imbalance. When we set ourselves apart from the environment, we may forget the healing effects of time spent in nature.

When we lose contact with fresh air, clean water, green earth, and sunshine, we get sick. This is not sentiment or romanticism. It is a demonstrable truth. As one example, consider what is known as seasonal affective disorder (SAD). This is a form of depression caused by a lack of full-spectrum light (like light from the sun). People with this disorder become seriously depressed during winter months, when there is not enough sunshine, particularly in northern regions. And while the full-blown version of this disorder is rare, it demonstrates in dramatic fashion a truth about all of us. We all need the sunshine. We all have a tendency to be happier in the months of long daylight. Likewise, suicide rates are higher during the months of short daylight.

Desert Plants Belong in the Desert

When we experience ourselves as distinct from the environment, we take on the role of choreographer or art critic. We want to alter and improve nature rather than enjoy it. Sometimes when Beverly and I sit in our backyard, we find ourselves busy with plans to improve what we see—the grass needs to be mowed, some weeds need to be pulled, the fence needs repair. We have to smile at our busy minds and come back to the present moment and enjoy sitting in our yard. Because not all our efforts are true improvements. Isn't our natural landscape—our forests and mountains, our lakes and rivers—perfect without our alterations? In an effort to get close to this beauty, we are tempted to "improve" it by building homes and resorts. But these destroy the very thing we admire.

Here in New Mexico, we enjoy the distinctive beauty of the desert landscape. But the desert is by no means untouched. People have brought in all kinds of vegetation inconsistent with a desert climate and the scarcity of water. We have replaced native plants, which survived with little attention, with non-natives that require lots of care and much scarce and precious water.

We visited a friend's home recently, and he commented on the desert plants he had just put in his yard. He said that he and his wife had come full circle in their landscaping efforts. Years ago, they had replaced desert vegetation with shrubs and grass that require frequent watering. Over the years they gradually progressed to landscaping that is more consistent with the New Mexico climate. Recently, they xeriscaped their whole backyard, which was now suspiciously reminiscent of some of their original natural vegetation.

As we all accept ourselves as part of the natural environment, we become more cautious about improving the natural beauty of our world. Without mindfulness of the unity of our own lives with nature, many of the alterations we impose upon our environment risk creating a life-threatening imbalance for our planet.

A Spiritual Awakening

In *Walden*, Henry David Thoreau described how he set out to live in the woods with only the barest of necessities for survival. He thought it most important that we pare down to those things which are absolutely crucial for human life. What are life's essentials? Do we need pots and pans? Well, only a few. A bed, blankets, a change of clothing, a small cabin, some basic food—there are few things required for a basic human life. He examined all that we regularly purchase, consume, and collect with an eye toward whether each item was indispensable. Could we live without it? Was it necessary for survival? Would we perish without this item?

Even in his time, Thoreau saw that while civilization continued to improve our houses, it did little to improve the people living in them. With prophetic clarity, he saw the vicious cycle of working to ensure more comforts, getting used to this level of comfort to the point of seeing it as a necessity, and then increasing the time spent working to afford these new comforts.

Thoreau sought more than an itemized list of necessities for human survival. He sought nothing less than a spiritual awakening by returning to a simple, basic life, unencumbered by society's demands or by modern conveniences and distractions. He suggested that we simplify our lives and quit the merry-go-round, and return to our essentially spiritual nature. He taught that feeding our souls must take priority and is critical for human survival.

PRACTICE

Shop for True Necessities

As a consciousness-raising device, make at least one grocery shopping trip in which you allow yourself to purchase only what you really need to live. Make a bargain with yourself that you will have to come back, making a special trip for items you really miss but that are not truly necessary.

Some of the obvious things we don't need:

- prepared foods and instant meals
- soft drinks
- the many variations of cleaning supplies
- snacks and desserts

A lot of other things may appear to be somewhere in between a true necessity and a convenience. You have to decide which they are. But if you do this exercise with some mindfulness, you will be surprised at how few things end up in your shopping cart. You may never view grocery shopping in quite the same way.

Reinventing Play

Most of us are not trotting off into the woods to live apart from civilization, nor should we. We'd ruin the woods. But we can consider how we spend our recreational time. Do we make adequate provision for experiencing our unity with nature? Do we care for the bit of nature around us? Do we care for the bit of nature that is our own body?

There are no hard and fast rules that apply uniformly to all of us. Three hours of jogging per week may be fabulous for one person, while three thirty-minute walks feel just right to another. Some of us love cross-country skiing, while others enjoy hiking. Communing in nature for some individuals will not necessarily require exercising in nature. Simply being outdoors and allowing nature into one's life may suffice.

You might wish to keep a recreational journal for a week or two. Make a note of time spent in recreational activities. Note also how you feel afterward, rating your sense of well-being following each activity from 1 to 10. This is a clear, concise way of determining how much time you truly spend in nature, how much time you spend in activities that you enjoy, and how much time is allotted to passive activities that don't really restore you. With this record in hand, you can ask:

> Am I satisfied with one hour of walking per week?
> Do I want to spend more time hiking?
> Is ten hours per week of television viewing more time than I intend to set aside for passive entertainment?
> Are there enough regular scenic trips in my schedule?
> Do I find that I live close to the ocean but rarely get there to enjoy it?
> Are the mountains just a scenic backdrop while I drive around the city?

The most important reason for examining how we spend our leisure time is not to berate ourselves, but to nourish ourselves, to make more conscious choices, to ensure that we spend our precious life moments in a satisfying and healing way. The chances are good that if you examine your leisure time activities closely, you will discover that many are not as satisfying as you think.

Another possible intervention is to pick one or two activities that you feel you spend too much time on and contract with yourself to eliminate or substantially reduce at least one unwanted leisure activity for one week. It may be passive time spent watching television that you wish to cut out of your schedule for a week's trial. Perhaps you would like to put a hold on shopping for a week, or eliminate card games that you have determined take up too much leisure time.

Of course, it is important for people in early recovery to refrain from activities associated with their addiction. Unfortunately, this may need to include some otherwise wonderful outdoor recreation. Many of us here in New Mexico enjoy fishing in our mountain streams and lakes. But if fishing has a strong association with drinking—as it does for some people—they may need to skip fishing until they have established some solidity in their new way of being. But early recovery is a perfect time for assessing and altering time spent in activities that do not employ your higher human capacities. Rather than merely give up a past destructive activity, such as drinking in the neighborhood bar, and rely on willpower only, it may be a useful practice to examine how you spend your precious time on earth.

Exercising Outdoors

You may choose to increase time spent exercising for the resulting health benefits, or perhaps to lose some unwanted pounds. Exercising will keep your body healthier, increase your sense of well-being, and improve your state of mind. Some of you may choose to exercise purely for the joy of exercising, while others may add walking or jogging to your schedules to stay fit and to improve upon your general health. These are fabulous reasons for exercising, and adding exercise into your recreational schedule will have very beneficial results. But please consider the added benefits of exercising outdoors, not just exercising for the benefits of exercise. That stationary bicycle you have inside may exercise your muscles, but it does little to feed your spirit. Mindfulness teaches us to enjoy the moment, not just the results.

Walking outdoors in a natural setting provides you with additional benefits from your walking meditation. While walking, you have the opportunity to be mindful of the trees and the magnificent blue sky. You may mindfully enjoy the birds and the animals you pass. You can choose a beautiful setting as your destination, such as a lake, a beach, the mountains, or the forest, and be mindful of your breathing while walking to your special place in nature. Try saying, "Beautiful!" over to yourself as you breathe in and out and walk, using the word to bring you into contact with the many beautiful aspects of nature. Even ordinary neighborhoods offer beautiful natural elements to enjoy; if there are no trees or flowers, there is always the sky.

Mindful awareness of each step taken in nature centers you, in addition to providing exercise. Being mindful of the breath while paying attention to and releasing your random thoughts back into the universe heightens your awareness and appreciation of nature. You become able to see your surroundings. Watch the cat leap the fence with grace and ease. Notice how the dogs alert one another to your approach, calling to their friends in neighboring yards. See each bird as the most precious being you ever saw. Allow the fragrance of the flowers to reach you. Attune yourself to the signs of the changing seasons, the changing rhythms of sunrise and sunset, the phases of the moon.

In bad weather a treadmill or a stationary bike will provide the opportunity to exercise. But it's a poor substitute for walking in a meadow or hiking up a mountain. We may receive the same physical benefits, but we miss out on the beauty and peacefulness a walk in nature has to offer. We will have exercised, but missed a chance to feed our souls.

If you live in the city, meadows and mountains may be hours away. But you can always notice the elements of nature that are available, such as the blue sky or grey clouds, or a tree planted here or there. You might like to make a special intention to regularly visit places where you can touch the natural world—a park, a zoo, an aquarium, a botanical garden, or an arboretum. And since most cities were established along important waterways, you can also visit the river or bay or ocean, walking along any promenades near the water or even taking a boat ride when you can. For that matter, even a baseball stadium can provide a comforting sight of green grass and open space, and this may be part of our attraction to such places to begin with. And of course, whenever you can, do your best to leave the city now and then. Certainly don't let years go by without visiting nature.

Renewal

The word *recreation* is a beautiful, important word. We seldom consider its true meaning—to refresh, restore, renew ourselves, to re-create, to become like new. Most of what we blithely call recreation is no such thing. While there is nothing evil per se about watching television or playing video games, we are not re-created or nourished by such activities.

When you walk, you may wish to choose a place in nature that you return to over and over again for a source of comfort, pleasure, or inspiration. You may walk, jog, hike, or bike to that special natural setting. You may prefer to meditate outdoors upon reaching your destination, or you may enjoy just sitting and taking it all in. This place may be a place to think, make decisions, mull over choices, and work out life problems.

When you meditate while sitting on a cliff at the ocean, or on a rock in the mountains, you may experience increased oneness with nature. The artificial division between you and the natural environment falls away. You come more into harmony with the natural world, and by doing so, you also come into harmony with yourself. For you are a walking, talking, breathing, thinking part of the natural world. If you become more centered, more tuned in to your natural rhythms, this carries over into the rest of your activities. You may be able to hold on to the centeredness and bring it with you into your work. You may discover a shift in you interactions with friends, family, or coworkers.

At home, you can use these experiences as the basis for visualizations of your special place even while sitting in your living room. Close your eyes, take deep breaths, and go on an imaginary journey to your beautiful setting in nature. Even when you cannot venture out to this beautiful destination, you may be able to reap similar meditative benefits by taking yourself on a guided journey there.

Protecting and Nurturing Yourself

In *New Seeds of Contemplation* (1961) Trappist monk Thomas Merton wrote about contemplation and recollection, words akin to our practice of minduflness:

> Do everything you can to avoid the noise and the business of men. Keep as far away as you can from the places where they gather to cheat and insult one another, to exploit one another, to laugh at one another, or to mock one another with their false gestures of friendship. Be glad if you can keep beyond the reach of their

radios. Do not bother with their unearthly songs. Do not read their advertisements.

The contemplative life certainly does not demand a self-righteous contempt for the habits and diversions of ordinary people. But nonetheless, no man who seeks liberation and light . . . can afford to yield passively to all the aspects of a society of salesmen and consumers. . . .

Keep your eyes clean and your ears quiet and your mind serene. Breathe God's air. Work, if you can, under His sky.

But if you have to live in a city and work among machines and ride in the subways and eat in a place where the radio makes you deaf with spurious news and where the food destroys your life and the sentiments of those around you poison your heart with boredom, do not be impatient, and accept it as the love of God and as a seed of solitude planted in your soul. If you are appalled by those things, you will keep your appetite for the healing silence of recollection.

Do what you can to take hold of your time, each precious moment of your life. Break the cycle that requires special, enhanced experiences of entertainment, which are so often also connected with substance abuse. Learn to treasure even the frustration of being cooped up in cars and offices away from earth, water, and sky, hearing this very frustration as a call to return to the natural world. You are that natural world, and it is you.

Doorway Six

LOVING

When you plant lettuce, if it does not grow well, you don't
blame the lettuce. You look into the reasons it is not doing
well. It may need fertilizer, or more water, or less sun. Yet if
we have problems with our friends or our family, we blame
the other person. But if we know how to take care of them,
they will grow well, like lettuce. Blaming has no positive
effect at all, nor does trying to persuade using reason and
arguments. . . . No blame, no reasoning, no argument, just
understanding. If you understand, and you show that you
understand, you can love, and the situation will change.
  —Thich Nhat Hanh, *Peace Is Every Step* (1991)

∞

*Cultivate healthy relationships to discourage addiction. Many people
become addicted in part because of painful and unsatisfying relationships. In turn, addiction can destroy even the best relationship. As
you become more mindful of relationship patterns, you can begin to
change them, reducing the need to indulge your addiction.*

∞

When people stop using, they are often at a loss as to how to
develop healthy relationships, improve existing ones, and
abandon hurtful or growth-stunting ways of interacting
with others. This is an important learning process because healthy,

loving, relationships help guard against a return to an addictive lifestyle. As Yogi Amrit Desai of Kripalu used to say, "Company is stronger than willpower." Healthy relationships with healthy people inoculate us against many problems. People who have a network of supportive relationships are healthier and happier than those who do not.

The literature on codependent relationships places too much emphasis on labeling and blaming, but it does underscore the lack of healthy, supportive, empowering relationships with individuals who overindulge in alcohol or drugs. How does an alcoholic ever come to see the people in his life honestly, without distortion or embellishment? How does Mary cope when she is angered by or disappointed with her partner? How does Harry deal with coming home to young children running wild? Generally, drugs and alcohol are used to escape life problems and create distance in relationships. Even when not flagrantly in evidence, the substance disorder lurks in the background, so that partners of people with substance abuse problems are constantly reacting to, guarding against, or angry about their partner's problem.

When Beverly stopped smoking many years ago, the removal of the smokescreen of cigarettes caused her to reexamine her friendships. She had become accustomed to stifling feelings and creating protective walls by reaching for a cigarette. With cigarettes out of her life, the protective walls dissolved and she was left to face the reality of her emotions and her relationships. A long process of change ensued.

When we leave addiction behind, we need to learn how to love ourselves and others all over again.

Relationships

Two basic human tendencies that complicate our relationships to others are our habit of seeing things only from our own point of view, and related to this, our tendency to blame. We see other people as either furthering our needs or frustrating them. When they meet our needs, they are blameless; when they don't, they are blameworthy. This is natural and understandable. At the same time, to have healthy relationships we must be able to go beyond this narrow view and see people for who they are in themselves, not just in terms of how they affect us.

The people in our lives are the plants in our garden. Take a look at them. How are they doing? How are your major relationships faring?

PRACTICE

See It from Their Perspective

On a piece of paper or in your journal, list the names of the people who are most important in your life, including, as appropriate, your partner, your closest friends, and your closest family members. Beginning with the first person on your list, breathe gently and consciously in and out. Let yourself become one with this person, feeling her feelings, feeling her life as your own life. Take your time. Then imagine her speaking to you about what her life is like and how it is to have a relationship with you. Write it all down, including all that is good and all that is less than good. If it feels appropriate, you might like to take the additional step of checking out your insight with the other person at an opportune time. Do this with each person on your list.

How is your human garden faring?

If you are fortunate, many of these relationships bring a smile to your face when you consider them. But if you are honest with yourself, most likely some of these relationships are complicated and painful in some way. Chances are, when you think about the painful aspects of your relationships, you will evoke one of two kinds of mental tapes: either a lot of mental chatter blaming the other person for the problems and justifying your own reactions, or else a lot of chatter about what an awful person you are. Worst of all, you can have both sorts of tape running at the same time.

If you are a gardener, you know that even gardens can evoke feelings of guilt or blame. If your lettuce is not doing well, you can get caught up in either blaming yourself ("I should have watered more often. I should not have let the weeds grow like that.") or blaming external factors ("These were not very good seeds. They are not very hardy plants."). And again, you can have both of these happening at the same time. But neither blaming ourselves or someone else is helpful. Both leave us alienated, angry, sad, and isolated.

Giving, Not Giving In

The central problem in all relationships is, *How can I give without giving in? How can I change, without losing myself?* Therapists have many techniques to help couples with this difficulty—listening skills, speaking skills, assertiveness. But more important than the techniques is what the techniques aim it—helping people see themselves and their partners in a new way. They aim at helping create a sense of "we-ness" out of which one operates, instead of a sense of alienation or "me against you." The sense of *giving in* to the other and sacrificing our own needs must be converted to a sense of *giving to* the relationship, or no technique will suffice.

The sense of we-ness is not something that can just be created intellectually, though you can describe it at that level. The tools therapists use aim at helping people have a new kind of *experience*—an experience of a we instead of a struggle. If people stay locked in competition or blame or guilt, there is no experience of we. But where you can create the experience of we, and insofar as you create this experience, alienation and struggle cease. For there is a fundamental antagonism between these two psychological states. To the extent you are experiencing things on the level of "we are in this together," you are not experiencing things as "I have to protect my own interests."

Guilt and shame are a flow of negative energy toward oneself. Anger and blame, on the other hand, are a flow of negative energy toward others. But both have a basic similarity: both prevent healing. In both cases, you are not attending to what needs doing. While you are feeling guilty about the watering you didn't do, and while you are angry about the poor quality of your seeds, you are not taking care of your lettuce. Both are an attempt to reduce our distress by understanding the situation and creating some sense of order out of the chaos of our experience. But both are destructive. Both prevent change.

The way to give without giving in is to create a different kind of experience. The way to change without losing yourself is to come from a different place, the place where you experience less separation between you and other. But how do you get to that place of knowing our interconnectedness, to the sense of we? To understand how to do this, we must first take a closer look at what gets in the way.

Sometimes when I work with couples, there is a very simple question on my mind: Why don't they just give each other what they want? Of course, in a way this is very naïve. There are many reasons why people do not give the other what is wanted. But perhaps the greatest obstacle is a feeling of losing, a feeling that giving is giving in, a fear of being taken advantage of without being given consideration in return. Sometimes we say this is a communication problem, as if the people involved do not know what the other wants. And occasionally, that even may be the case. But with most couples in conflict, they know all too well what the other wants. They are just not willing to give it.

Perhaps Susan would like you to call her now and then. Perhaps George would like you to appreciate the quality of his thinking. Maybe your son needs you to just enjoy being with him. Maybe your wife would like you to turn off the television when she comes in and notice her. Of course, you do not have to do these things.

But why not?

The *first* one to benefit from this practice will be you.

All My Dreams Fulfill

Plato tells the ancient myth—ancient even in his day—of soul mates. At some time way back, in the time of the beginning, there were three kinds of beings: male-male, female-female, and male-female. These beings were tragically split apart, and then spent a good portion of their subsequent lives trying to find their other halves and rejoin them. This story speaks to us as strongly today as it did to ancient women and men. It even has a modern tone in allowing that not all opposite halves are of the opposite gender. Most of us can easily resonate with this yearning for another to complete us. Many have a sense of finding their opposite halves in another person, of having—or at least wanting—a soul mate. This is a real and precious phenomenon—one of the most wonderful things in life.

Yet this same idea, if taken in an unexamined, literal way, can become an obstacle to finding and keeping good relationships. When

Elvis sings plaintively of his desire to be loved tender, to be loved true, so far so good. But when he asks the other to fulfill all his dreams, we must pause. This may be wonderful romantic poetry. But as a life story—as an expectation, concretely and literally, of what the romantic partner should do for us—it is a disaster. No one can fulfill all our dreams. No matter how wonderful the relationship, it cannot be.

Intellectually most people would probably agree that one should not literally expect fulfillment from another person. But this is a deeper matter than the words we speak. At the level of myth and story, at an emotional level, we may still act out of this kind of expectation. Every generation since the troubadours has had its love songs and poetry, whether it's Old Blue Eyes, Elvis, or the Beatles. This stuff seeps in through our pores, soaks deep down into the psyche, persuading us that some other person is supposed to come along and make everything right.

Exalted notions of romantic love have other effects. For one thing, they devalue other kinds of relationships. In this spirit, Thomas Moore in his book, *Soul Mates* (1994), refuses to limit the concept to romantic partners. Can't a friend be a soul mate as well? A parent, a child, a brother or sister, a teacher or student? Restricting soul mate status to romantic couples diminishes these other relationships, according them secondary status and intensifying the loneliness of those who are without partners.

Most of us remain devoted to the ideal of romantic love. Nothing in life hurts more, yet nothing is more wonderful either. It is wonderful to have someone to love, and someone to share the day-to-day stuff with. Having love in your life gives you a radiant center, which can suffuse everything with a sense of calm and stability. Yet if on some emotional level we are expecting another to make everything wonderful and easy, we are loading that relationship with an impossible burden of expectation.

Cinderella and Prince Charming

It is this overexpectation that explains why everywhere men and women are angry at each other. Even today's liberated women have undertones of Cinderella and other fairy tales at their core, a fantasy that some prince will sweep them off their feet, and everything from then on will be wonderful and easy, living "happily ever after." And the only qualification for this bliss—the only thing you need to do to earn this—is have the shoe fit. But when they discover that Prince Charming has needs and flaws and weaknesses of his own, it is a bitter disappointment, the source of much grief and anger. Even in our supposedly more enlightened time, many little girls are still being raised with a focus on their wedding day as the pinnacle of their lives. It is no wonder that they are then entirely unprepared for the life with a flesh-and-blood man that follows.

As difficult as this situation is for women, the situation for men may be worse in the sense that male expectations are even less accessible to awareness. Little boys are given complex messages about love. On the one hand, they are still instructed that the unpardonable sin for a man is to have needs. Men are supposed to be somehow above all that. And yet, being mere mortals, the needs are nonetheless there. In fact, under the principle that what is denied gains power, these needs can be even stronger for having been driven underground. The message to little boys is a complex one, and a difficult story line to fulfill. Men are supposed to be a James Bond or Clint Eastwood character, always capable, always knowing what to do, never needy. Yet just under the surface lie deep needs—much of which somehow are supposed to be taken care of by the women in their lives. The need to be admired, to be cared for, to be seen as attractive, and other needs are even stronger and more difficult to work with because they are less accessible in men. Where male neediness does emerge, however, is under stress. When men are sick, see what happens to the veneer of rigid strength. And when men get divorced, they are often unprepared for how difficult it is for them emotionally.

To be out of touch with what we need is not to be mindful. When we do not even know what it is we need from the people in our lives, we certainly cannot ask them for it, or even examine whether our needs are reasonable. Yet when these unconscious needs are unfulfilled, the relationship can take on a quality of seething resentment without our even knowing why.

Some men try valiantly to keep their needs hidden. Unfortunately, some succeed all too well. When this happens, their partners may completely believe their myth of brittle strength, and even find it hard to imagine them needing anything. This was the case with Jennie and her husband, for example. Jennie was in therapy at the beginning of midlife. For years, Jennie had hidden her feelings about her marriage in a bottle. But when she stopped drinking, Jennie found she was furious with her police officer husband. He had utterly failed to live up to his self-advertised strong, independent male image. She was enraged at him for not taking care of her as she had assumed he would. Beneath the anger, she was also deeply sad and disappointed in their marriage, and scared about the future. This was not the story she wanted to write for her life. He was supposed to save her from her family, take care of her, make it a happily-ever-after life story. When after weeks of exploring Jennie's disappointment, grief, and anger, I began to gently suggest that perhaps her husband had needs, too, Jennie was incredulous. It had never seriously occurred to her that men need anything. Still less had it occurred to her that men might need anything from women, or that her husband might need anything from her. This idea was glaringly out of sync with her own myths about men and women— so much so that she dropped out of therapy after that. If Jennie does not become more mindful of this pattern, she will probably continue to be with men who exude an outer strength, but who eventually disappoint her.

This profound anger and disappointment between romantic partners explains the incredible and persistent popularity of books on the subject of relationships—especially those which tell us that men are like this and women are like that. In one way, such books are inevitably an oversimplification of the problem. We may recognize ourselves to some extent in these pages, but it is a distorted and stereotyped reflection. And we find ourselves reading these books with a running commentary: "Yes, I do that. Yes, my partner is like that. But this idea only fits a little. And we're not like that at all."

Falling in Love

Jungian psychology throws a helpful light on this problem. According to Jung, men have an unconscious feminine aspect, which he calls the anima, and women an unconscious masculine aspect, the animus. The ecstasy of falling in love is a process of projection, the man projecting his unintegrated feminine side onto a woman, the woman projecting her unintegrated masculine side onto the man. That is why there is indeed a sense of the other person completing us. For through this process of projection, we activate our own unconscious half.

The problem is that no real-life woman can adequately embody the anima, as no real-life man can embody the animus. There is a contradiction contained in this process of falling in love. We say we love these people, but then we expend an incredible amount of energy trying to get them to be what they're supposed to be, instead of trying to see and nurture who they really are. For it is not the other person we are really seeing, but the desired animus or anima, our own rejected other side. Such love can quickly change into bitterness, anger, and hatred.

Yet the heart of the problem is simple: we expect too much. We have such unrealistic expectations of our partners that *we do not see them as people in their own right, but entirely in terms of our own needs and expectations.* The real solution, therefore, has less to do with understanding that when women say this they mean that, and that men are this way because of that (though this can help somewhat), but to begin to *see the other person for his or her own sake.*

Seeing others clearly can be difficult. And then, of course, if you take two people who are enraged at each other due to a profound disappointment of fundamental expectations, and you throw alcohol or some other drug onto these flames, a painful and difficult situation easily becomes a conflagration. Not only has this man not turned out to be her Prince Charming, but he's a drunk besides. And when he drinks, he ignores her and says unkind things. Through the warm but distorted glow of alcohol, he sees his bar mates as the people who really understand him, whom he can say anything to because he feels so close to them—until he actually presumes too much and risks coming to blows. But all that, of course, is forgotten in the next intoxicated glow of pseudofriendship.

In alcoholic-partner relationships, one of the most common dances is that of control/rebel. The more she controls, the more he feels his freedom threatened. And the more threatened his freedom, the more he rebels. At the same time, the more he rebels, the more she feels unsafe and needs to control. The more upset she gets when he stays out late drinking, the more he needs to assert his freedom by doing just that. People trapped in this dance may even sense how trapped they are, and how ineffective their repeated responses are to these situations. But they feel as though they can't help it.

Teachers and Students

It is not only romantic relationships that suffer from unexamined expectations. Other relationships do as well. One example is the teacher-student relationship. There are millions of teachers in the world, but very few mentors. A mentor is that special person who can see and nurture the possibilities in the student. The mentor is the ideal teacher, the archetypal teacher. But not all teachers can be mentors, and even those who are cannot be mentors to everyone. So what happens in most teacher-student relationships—even in the best of them—is that the teacher tries to find students who already reflect to some degree the ideas the teacher holds, and then molds the student to make her ideas increasingly resemble the teacher's.

On the other side, when students have too idealized a view of teachers, they expect teachers to give things that they do not have to give, while refusing to accept the gifts the teachers actually possess. This also occurs between parents and children, with parents not seeing the child's individual and special nature and cultivating that, but trying to make the child over in the parents' image. And few children grow up enough to see their parents as people with their own needs and their own dreams, and not just an oppressive force to fight against or escape from.

The way out of these destructive patterns is to begin to focus on the real person instead of seeing the other only as a symbol of our frustrated needs and unfulfilled, impossible longings.

Seeing the Other

When was the last time you really *saw* your partner, your child, your friend? We can get so caught up in what we want from them or fear from them, that we never really see them. And by this we mean, first of all, literally *seeing*, just taking in the visual gestalt of the other person. Seeing with compassion begins with simply seeing. As a Buddhist sutra says in a literal translation: "compassionate eyes seeing living beings."

When we come home from work, anxious to tell our stories of success or struggle, can we actually take a moment first, slow down, and see each other—take in the other person as he or she is in that moment and not just as the person exists in our imagination? Your partner is the flower of your garden. How is she doing? Does he look fresh and thriving? Or is he starting to droop a little? What does she need? What does he need?

To begin with, do not even try to do anything about any of this. Just look. Just practice seeing. Our partner is our flower, but sometimes we are afraid to see how our flowers are doing. Because then we might feel burdened by having to do something about it. And we don't want to. We are too busy wanting them to change to suit our needs and ideal image. So start simply with the act of seeing. You do not need to do anything you do not want to do or are not ready to do. Just look. Check in. See what is actually there. Perhaps you will begin to experience a softening, an opening of the heart that will allow you to do something helpful, without feeling as though you are giving in.

PRACTICE

See Each Other at Meals

In too many households, meals are no longer a time of coming together. Make it a practice to share at least one meal with each other daily. Turn the television off. Let the answering machine take care of the phone. As you sit down to eat, breathe in and out a few times, enjoying the prospect of the food, making eye contact and smiling at each other. Once a week or so, conduct an entire meal in silence. *See* each other.

Hearing Deeply

When was the last time you listened deeply to another person? As therapists, we know this is difficult. By the nature of therapy, clients are not friends—at least not in the usual sense. They are not people you socialize with. Therapy is set up this way because it is easier to listen deeply to people who are outside of the rest of our lives, where their needs and expectations may otherwise be in conflict with our own. When others' needs and expectations are in conflict with our own, these things get in the way of being able to hear deeply.

A therapist must be able to put aside his own reactions, and this is not always easy. A client of mine once spoke angrily about city leash laws, because he likes to let his dogs be off leash. He spoke strongly against the intolerance of non–dog owners. Tapes started playing in my head. On the one hand, I'd had dogs, too, and loved to let them be as free as possible. On the other hand, I'd been chased a few too many times by dogs when I used to jog. I'd had a few too many dog owners say sweetly, "Oh, he won't bite," as their adored pet approached, growling and baring its teeth.

Both the part of me that agreed and the part that disagreed with the client's opinion about leash laws made it hard to hear the person. What I needed to do was put my opinion aside for the moment, and hear what this person was telling me—feeling the loneliness beneath the opinion, knowing how important these animals were to him for love and companionship. And then I could understand. *To understand, it is not necessary to agree.*

Now with our friends or family, how often do we do that? We all too readily load up the tape of our opinions, instead of taking in deeply what the other person has to say and the meaning behind the communication. Granted, in nontherapy relationships you may want to express your feelings about irresponsible pet owners as well. But do we have to do that in knee-jerk fashion, without hearing the other person out? Can we first give her some room to air her feelings before we express our own?

A therapist may be the only person in someone's life who is willing to hear him out without just reacting—without just loading up a prerecorded tape of ready-made opinions. This is one of the main reasons we are a society that needs therapists. With shifts in the nature of therapy today, and with economic pressures from managed health care, even therapists are less likely to actually give the person room to let out what she needs to say and to take it in deeply and nonjudgmentally. We would be a healthier society if we could learn to do this for each other.

Holding Opinions Loosely

There is a Buddhist teaching that we should not hold on to our views and opinions too tightly—not even Buddhist ones. This is very important when it comes to being a loving person. If we make our opinions and views a barrier between us and other people, we are emphasizing what divides us rather than the common experience of being human. Yet the common experience of being human is so much more essential and fundamental.

Sometimes we think choosing friends is a matter of finding people who view things in the same way. "If you view things the same way I do, then you can become a friend. If not, this is not possible." By this standard, very few people can become friends, and even among those, very few can remain friends. Because at some point, you always discover important ways in which the other's point of view differs from your own.

Even more seriously, tightly held views contain a seed of violence. When people wage war for property and possessions, that is bad enough. But people who are seeking property and possessions will not destroy as they wage war; otherwise, what have they gained? It is the ideologues who are dangerous when waging war. They wage war for an idea, and because of this idea, are willing to kill and destroy without mercy.

Hold your opinions lightly. Many of your most cherished beliefs contain at least some error, no matter how insightful you are. Do not let your views come between you and other people.

Active Listening

One thing we can all do in order to hear others better is something quite simple. It is called "active listening." On the surface, active listening is simply restating or paraphrasing what the other person has said. But that is just the external aspect of this practice. Active listening is a deep practice, a practice of openness to the point of view and experience of the other person. It requires you to temporarily set aside your own point of view to make space for the other person.

Why should you paraphrase what someone else says? A full explanation would take us deep into communication theory. But in essence, it is important because it shows your intention to understand, and because it prevents miscommunication.

Here is an actual verbal exchange the two of us had one day driving in the car:

Beverly: "How long have you had this tape in the tape deck?"

Tom: "Oh, about a week I guess."

Most women will understand that what Beverly was really asking was, "Could we please change this tape? I'm sick of it." Many men, on the other hand, would think that I had answered the question properly. For one thing, this is one of those areas where women and men communicate differently. Women tend to ask for things a little indirectly, avoiding putting the other person on the spot. But more importantly for present purposes, this exchange demonstrates that even when you think the message you are sending is unambiguously clear and direct, it may not be clear to the other person.

Now this is a trivial case, of course, and it was easily resolved. But what if you are not just talking about the musical selection, but are discussing something with real emotional sensitivity attached to it? Then you cannot afford a misunderstanding. Taking the time to paraphrase what the other has said can prevent a lot of misunderstandings. It is an act of deep respect for the other person and the importance of his or her communication.

There are many theories about why doing this seemingly simple thing is so helpful. But we like best the way Carl Rogers—the psychologist who first described this approach—came to talk about it. After years of complex theorizing about it, near the end of his career Rogers came to say that what he was doing in reflective listening was simply *checking his understanding* of what the other person was saying. This keeps the focus for the listener where it should be: on simply trying to understand the other person.

Like all deep practices, active listening must not be done mechanically. The outer form of paraphrase needs to be backed up with an open heart and a sincere intention to understand. When this happens, it is very pleasant to be listened to in this way. You can feel how much the other person wants to understand. Instead of *telling* us that we are important and valued, they *show* us.

Avoid Mixed Messages

A lot of things can contaminate this process. If a slightly sarcastic tone of voice creeps into the reflection, it can communicate that you are not checking your understanding at all, but are really pointing out how silly the other person's communication is. Or if you perfectly mirror what the other person said, but you are staring at your watch or jangling your car keys, the other person may accurately perceive that you are not interested in understanding her. And some people cannot resist throwing in their own opinions or changing the subject, thinking they are doing reflection:

"You said so-and-so, but that's wrong!"

"You shouldn't look at it that way!"

"Well, you said you feel badly about it, but I think . . ."

"I know just what you mean. It's just like what happened to me the other day. . . ."

These responses are not wrong. They could conceivably even be helpful sometimes. But they are not listening. If you stay close to the simple spirit of the thing—trying to deeply understand the other without judgment, and actively checking your understanding of the other person—you will not be far off. This is a wonderful gift to give another person. It is sunshine and water and fertilizer for your lettuce, all in one.

PRACTICE

Listen Deeply

The next time someone you care about is speaking to you about something of some importance, take a deep breath. Calm your mind for the moment. Still your own opinions and reactions for now. (You'll get back to them later.) Don't step on the ends of his sentences the moment he seems to be done, but pause. Be sure he has finished. Drink in deeply what he has said, and give him space to express it fully. And don't just hear, but listen. Actively. Reflectively. Wonderful things can happen.

The Absence of Touch May Be Hazardous to Your Health

There are famous studies in developmental psychology that demonstrate the necessity of touch for infants. Babies in an orphanage were assigned at random to either receive a lot of touch and caressing, or the minimal touch they normally received at the institution. The results were striking. The babies who received touch were much healthier physically, cognitively, and emotionally than those who did not. Babies who were not touched often showed "failure to thrive" syndrome and did not grow as they should have, or even died.

Touching, then, is a vital area of human life. It is an area with incredible potential for healing. And it is an area with incredible potential for abuse. The whole area of touch must be healed so it can be used as an instrument of healing. In other words, it is an area of human life deeply in need of mindfulness. We need to be mindful of when we touch. And we need to be mindful of when we do not touch.

Given all the present-day complications surrounding touch in our litigious society, you must be very aware when you go about touching. Be aware of your intentions, and be sure you are not fooling yourself. Be aware of how you may be perceived, or misperceived, by the other person. Recognize any power differentials in the relationship. The greater the difference in power, the more caution is in order.

But in situations where you are clear, and where both you and the other person are open and ready, touching is a beautiful way of connecting. Do not let these moments pass without awareness. When your wife brushes her hand against yours, when your son places a hand on your shoulder, when you shake the hand of a friend, you can choose to let these be deep moments of connection.

Thich Nhat Hanh was initially at a loss when people wanted to hug him in this country. This was not a normal thing to a Buddhist monk from Southeast Asia. But by opening up to the experience, he even made it into a form of meditation. He advised that when you hold the other person, you breathe gently in and out, aware of your breath, aware of the other person, aware of yourself, aware of touching and of being touched. He even suggested using a gatha—a short poem used to encourage mindfulness—by telling yourself, "Breathing in, I know this person is alive in my arms. Breathing out, I am very happy." This way it becomes a deep practice.

We can easily underestimate the healing power of such a deceptively simple practice. What if you and the important people in your life made a conscious intention to hug each other this way whenever you part from each other or come back together? For one thing, it marks these as important moments in a relationship. It underscores the importance of the relationship, and gives you a chance to come out of the fog of mental chatter in which we too often live and experience the living, breathing reality of the people in your life.

Sexual Touch

Society is as neurotic about sex as it ever was. The form of the neurosis has changed, but the essence is the same. The sexual revolution, while seeming to offer greater freedom, was never truly integrated. It was excessive and naive to think that human beings could have such deep intimacy without responsibility, emotional involvement, and commitment. Given this excess, the predictable has happened. We have swung back in the direction of anxiety about sex and touching. The latest indication of this is the constant threat of litigation for touch in the workplace. On the one hand, of course, this is very important. Something had to be done to protect people who felt coerced to touch from those who had power over them. Yet the cost has been high. We have become even more paranoid and fearful in the whole area of sexuality and touch.

Even sex with our partners becomes overly goal oriented, fixated on genital pleasure and orgasm rather than appreciative of the whole sexual process. As an antidote for this and some of the problems it can cause, behavioral sex therapy developed something called *sensate focus*. When couples come in for therapy who are experiencing sexual difficulties, sensate focus is a technique to restore sexual functioning. Genital contact is made off limits for a time, while couples enjoy simply touching and being touched in nonerotic ways, such as massage. While practicing this kind of touch, each person focuses on the sensations involved, whether you are the giver or the receiver of the touching. The result is often that the barriers to sexual functioning are removed.

PRACTICE

Enjoy Mindful Touching

Set aside at least half an hour to practice mindful touch with your partner. Divide the time about in half between touching and being touched. Breathe mindfully. Practice touching and massaging the other person in gentle, nonsexual ways. When you are doing the touching, experience it as though you were the one being touched. And when you are receiving touch, imagine how it feels to be giving it. Close your eyes when possible in order to focus on the sensations, not trying to do anything or accomplish anything, just being present. Continue to breathe mindfully throughout. Share with each other what this experience was like.

Sensate focus is effective because it encourages people to refocus on the *process* rather than the goal. By learning to surrender to the here-and-now experience of touching and being touched, anxiety about performance and focus on the goal of orgasm no longer inhibit the natural flow. Does this sound a little like a mindfulness technique? It is.

If this approach is helpful to couples who are experiencing sexual dysfunction, perhaps it can be helpful to couples who are not as well. And not just because it may deepen your sexual life together, though this can certainly be a wonderful result. But perhaps even more importantly, because it can be a beautiful way to relate mindfully and sensually to each other, to deepen sensitivity to your partner, to deepen sensitivity to yourself, to reunify body and spirit. Besides all of which, it is just plain nice to do.

Living Things Need Space

One summer a few years ago, Beverly and I started gardening. This was a completely new experience for Beverly as a city person. And while I had done a little gardening a long time ago, we were both essentially novices. We knew we had to pay attention to spacing our rows adequately. Though we carefully read the directions on the seed packs, we still underestimated how much space our precious vegetables needed. And with a squeamishness laughable to seasoned gardeners, we hated thinning out the new young plants to allow sufficient room, and therefore often left plants growing too close together. Our clearest error, however, was with our tomato plants. We thought we had left lots of room, but by the end of the season, they had grown so big that that part of our garden was a small jungle. We could hardly find space to step between the plants in order to harvest our wonderful tomatoes.

All living things need space to grow and flourish. We need freedom; we need spiritual and emotional room.

Since theoretical physicists have wondered whether space and time are really different things, it is no longer strange to realize that sometimes the space we need is actually a need for time. In *Leaves of Grass* (1855) Whitman said that he loafed and invited his soul. And we all require some loafing and soul inviting to feel well, to be at home in our bodies and minds. It is hard to invite the soul when you are perpetually rushing from one thing to the next.

This is also very important with children. Many of us overschedule our children. They have no sense of spaciousness. They have no opportunity to learn to entertain themselves. When the balance between structured activity and free time is about right for our children, we may occasionally hear them say they are bored. Refrain from rushing in with a solution. See what they come up with themselves. Let them deal with the boredom. Boredom is an open space that is a little frightening because we don't quite know what to do with it at first. But as such, a little boredom is a teaching in disguise. It teaches us to be at home with some open space.

We also need emotional and mental space. When Beverly and I were novice therapists, we were very anxious to be helpful to our clients. We tried to do so by filling up all the space, trying to make helpful suggestions or interpretations, eliminating all uncomfortable silence. More and more we have come to believe in the therapeutic value of silent spaces. And when we rush in with an interpretation that is premature (if not plain wrong), we are crowding our client, not allowing him to discover something by himself.

You can do this with people outside the consulting room as well. Even if we mean well, and are trying to be attentive and loving, people need space to know what they are feeling, to discover what they want and need. They need space to experience their own thoughts and feelings before we intrude.

A friend told us how uncomfortable it can be for her when she visits her husband's family, because they are always asking her how she is and whether she needs anything. And while their solicitousness may be well intended, her in-laws hardly give her the chance to know what she is feeling before they see some intimation of it on her face and inquire about it. But part of being a good host is allowing your guest some space. Part of being a good parent, partner, therapist, teacher, or friend is also the art of allowing some space. True, at times there may be a fine line between allowing space and showing neglect or indifference. But most of the time it is not that hard to find the balance, if we focus on the need of the other person and not just on our own need to feel helpful.

To allow space, you must have peace in yourself. If you notice that your partner has a slight shadow over her face, it is not always best to jump on this right away and ask what is wrong. Sometimes when we ask too quickly, the other person becomes all the more entrenched in a negative mood state, because then she not only has a difficult mood to deal with, but our comments have made it more solid. We may be tempted to intervene in others' feelings out of insecurity, fearing that the other person is upset with us in some way. But as always, to be truly helpful to another person, we must first be truly helpful to ourselves. We have to take care of the insecure feeling in ourselves, rest in the strength of our relationship, and allow the other person space to feel what she is feeling. Perhaps she will decide on her own that she would like some deep listening about the problem. Of course, if she remains silent too long, we may get around to asking her very gently, very lovingly about this. But first we need to have peace and centeredness in ourselves so we do not end up adding to the difficulty.

Not Two

There is tremendous suffering and pain in the lives of addicted people. Oftentimes, the addiction itself is an attempt to avoid what hurts. But the addiction creates even more pain, both for the addicted individual and for the people around that person. It is easy to drown in this sea of hurt, suffering, and anger.

Psychologist Erich Fromm taught that *our capacity to love is a single capacity.* We do not have one capacity for loving others, and another capacity for loving ourselves. Our ability to love is one single ability. Insofar as we can be loving to ourselves, we can be loving to other people. Insofar as we can be loving to others, we can be loving to ourselves. Likewise, if we are hard on others, we are hard on ourselves, and if we are hard on ourselves, we are hard on others.

In this light, loving our neighbors as ourselves is not so much a commandment as it is a statement of psychological truth. The love with which we love the neighbor is ultimately the love with which we love ourselves, and vice versa. The measure you give is the measure you get back. Judge not that you be not judged. These teachings reveal that the level of openness, love, and understanding we have toward others is what we ourselves receive. And the level of love and understanding toward ourselves flows also toward others.

When we are critical of others, we express the same inner critic who criticizes us. When we are stingy with others, we are expressing our inner dragon, who hoards his treasure but does not know how to enjoy it. In doing so, we are directing this negative energy outward toward another person. But this same energy also comes back at us. We may be aware of some of the ways in which it comes back at us, or we may not know at all. But it always comes back. For at the deepest level, both psychologically and spiritually, we are deeply connected. We are one. (Or as the Buddhists would prefer to say, Not-Two).

Sometimes giving to others can feel unsafe. You might imagine that when you give, somehow you are diminished. And even though this is never ultimately the case, there can be an experience of fear attached to giving. For this reason, it is easier to begin by practicing love and generosity toward yourself. If you are loving and generous and wise with yourself, this attitude can begin to overflow toward your partner, your children, your parents, your friends, and your coworkers. And the most loving thing you can do for yourself is to learn to be with yourself as you really are.

A Healing Presence

When a baby cries, a loving mother does not come into the room and scold the baby for crying, saying, "What's the matter with you? Why don't you stop crying and grow up?" Yet when the little one in ourselves is crying, or angry and throwing a tantrum, or trembling with fear, this is often exactly the kind of message we give ourselves.

"What's the matter with you? You shouldn't feel hurt about this or worried about that. Grow up! Stop being a baby! That's life!"

The first step in being able to be a healing presence for others is to be a healing presence for ourselves. And the first step in being a healing presence to ourselves is the capacity to be with aspects of ourselves that we do not like, which hurt or cause shame. Like a loving mother, we must be able to be with these aspects of ourselves as with our own children.

If you have spent time with children, you know that children are very beautiful. But you also know they are not always easy. When they become tired or upset, they can try our patience deeply. And when they are difficult, we may not always want to be with them.

A female client with no children had a dream that expressed her ambivalence about them. In the dream, she finally got her beautiful baby. She was enjoying holding and cuddling the precious little infant. And then, when she had had enough, she simply put the baby away in a dresser drawer and went about her life. What makes this such a great dream is that it expresses so clearly the problem with children: they are *always* there. And no matter how much you love them, there are times when you just wish you did not have a child tugging at your sleeve, times when you are not ready for the "Mommy! Mommy! Daddy! Daddy! Look! Look!" The dream allowed this woman to have her cake and eat it, too—that is, to have her baby, but still be free.

But of course, good parents understand that children are a commitment. You cannot pick and choose the times when they will need you and the times when you would like to just have some peace and quiet. You must do your best to be there for them on their schedule, according to their needs, and not your own convenience. That is the nature of parenthood. Many of us complain about the failures of our parents, who were not sufficiently attuned to our needs in some way. But of course we cannot change that now. What we can do is learn to be good parents, beginning with ourselves. And that means parenting the most difficult parts of ourselves: the thoughts and feelings we least want. This is also the greatest gift to our children, and to all the people in our lives.

So when the people in your life are being their worst, their most difficult, their most demanding, it is time to remember that this is when they need you the most. This is when they need your love and acceptance and patience—not when it is easy because they are being pleasant. But you can only do this if you also practice parenting the difficult parts of yourself. When you know that you are tired, irritable, and difficult, this is the time you most need to give yourself understanding.

This is nothing abstract. The next time you get irritated, afraid, or feel sad—the next time you see a selfish or aggressive aspect of your personality surface—this is the very moment of healing. This is the time to breathe deeply, pause, and welcome these feelings. Embrace them. They are angels of mercy, opportunities for healing grace. By making a space in your life for these aspects of self, you kiss the frog and turn it into the handsome prince, you transform the base metals into gold. And the more you do this with yourself, the more you will be able to do this with the people in your life.

Interdependence

In the Buddhist Pali Canon there is a story about a father and daughter who made their living as acrobats. He would hold a long pole onto which she would climb up and perform stunts. The father realized how vulnerable they were. If anything happened to either one of them, they could not earn a living. So the father told the daughter that they must take good care of each other. You might say this was the codependent position. The daughter, however, disagreed. She said that what was important was that they each take care of themselves. When the father concentrates on holding his pole steadily, he is taking good care of himself. When the daughter performs her stunts mindfully, she is taking good care of herself. And it is by doing this that they also take care of each other.

The Buddha agreed with the daughter.

The choice ultimately is not between codependence and independence. Independence is at best a relative term. The deeper truth is that we are all *interdependent*. There is nowhere you can go where you are not vulnerable to the actions of other people. If you pack off to the most remote Himalayan cave, you are still affected by pollution and other consequences of human action. Likewise, when we take good care of ourselves, we are also taking good care of the people around us. When we take good care of our emotions, and learn to be loving and gentle with ourselves, there is nothing better that we could do for others. When we are not happy and peaceful, those around us suffer. And nothing helps the people we love more than for us to be happy and peaceful ourselves.

So loving others cannot be separated from loving ourselves, and loving ourselves cannot be separated from loving others. All of the approaches we discuss in this book—journaling, meditation, dreams, recreating, therapy—all of them are ways of recentering mindfully in our own lives. As the Zen story has it, the answer to the question of why the Bodhidharma—who brought Buddhism to China from India—came to the East is not some abstract reason, but the answer is, "Where are you?" That is, when you come back to yourself, to where you are and what is happening in the present, you come back to life. There is no more important thing that you can do for yourself, and nothing more important that you can do for anyone else.

We Are Never Separate

While studying in Europe one year, I met a student from Thailand. He taught me something very important, something that I have never forgotten. I was just nineteen years old, and while I had a wonderful year, there were also moments of deep loneliness being so far from home. I asked my friend, who had spent time as a Buddhist monk, if he did not get lonely as well. He smiled and said simply that whenever such feelings came to him, he looked around at the buildings and people, sensing the presence of these other beings, and then always knew he was not alone.

This connection is always available.

Doorway Seven

DREAMING

A myth is a public dream; a dream is a private myth.
—Joseph Campbell, *The Power of Myth*, 1988

❧

Explore dreams to expand your view of who you are beyond the limited point of view of your conscious, rational self. Dreams offer clues about what is missing and what is out of balance. Often these are blind spots which we have difficulty seeing consciously.

❧

When you are ill today, you go to the doctor—you visit the gleaming halls of medical science. But in the ancient world, you would have sought the healing of a god. In ancient Greece, for instance, you might have visited a temple of the divine healer Asklepios. When you arrived, the temple attendants would interview you, ensuring that the god had called you. For only those whom the god called would be accepted. If they determined he had called you, they would escort you to the inner sanctum to rest and await a dream. Should the god visit you in a healing dream, his attendants offered no interpretation; the dream was felt to be healing in itself.

If the problem for which you seek help today is addiction, you may be escorted into the halls of science rather than the sanctuary of

Asklepios. The sign of Asklepios, a serpent twirling around a staff, might still be in evidence. But chances are you would not notice it. Chances are, the physician would be equally unconscious of this silent invocation of the old god of healing. But he is there nonetheless. "Called or not," reads the Latin inscription over Carl Jung's door at his Bollingen retreat, "God will be present." At least half the power of the physician lies not in the science she practices, but in the silent, unconsciously invoked presence of the healing god.

Many today are no longer satisfied with the split between medical science and the spiritual. Our fascination with alternative medicine, while at times dangerously uncritical and naive, shows in part our need for a more integrative treatment, a treatment that includes the spiritual element. But every night, for those who have ears to hear, God speaks to us in a dream. One of the best things you can do to promote your own healing and wholeness is to begin to attend to these nightly messages.

Manny's Dream

I met Manny at a halfway house. Manny had been there about a month, following intensive inpatient treatment. He had been homeless for several years prior to that. Every so often he tried to make his way off the streets, but the next drinking binge would put an end to his attempt at reform. By this point, I had worked with many alcoholics. I was used to the vast quantities of alcohol some of them consumed. But when Manny told me how much he drank, I had to fight not to let my mouth drop open in amazement that the man before me was still alive.

Manny was not easy to get to know. Superficially friendly, he would greet me with a warm "Hey, Doc!" through a grin lacking several teeth. But beyond that, it was hard to get him to open up. Our meetings remained superficial. When I asked him about urges, he denied having any, acting as though it was a personal insult for me to think he might have had one. One day, he told me he had something important to say. He said he had had a dream last night. And in the dream, he had had a sip of whiskey. The whiskey had glowed and sparkled mysteriously. Drinking sent a surge of well-being through him.

It took a lot for Manny to tell me this. I knew he was worried that this meant something bad about him. I knew he feared it meant that he was about to relapse. I also knew I had to be careful. I could not plunge into deep dream interpretation with him without triggering a lot of fear. I could only tell him that this was a good dream, that it was safe and did not mean anything bad.

From what I knew of the program Manny was in, I guessed it had strengthened the idea in him that not only was drinking bad, but even having an urge to drink was bad, somehow reflecting a lack of resolve. Many of the patients I interviewed stalwartly refused to acknowledge any thoughts about drinking. They did not see how this attitude kept them trapped. Manny had repressed his awareness to such a point that his psyche was rebelling through this dream against the one-sidedness of his conscious self. If he had been able to, he might have acknowledged that he still had at times a desire to drink. With the dream leading the way, he could have learned to take care of these thoughts and feelings, rather than treat them with violence and repression. He might have found a way out of the struggle, the cycle of letting go into alcoholism, followed by clamping down, followed by another relapse.

What did Manny's dream mean? Since I did not have the chance to work it through with Manny, it is hard to say. On one level, it seemed obvious enough; Manny wanted a drink. And as much as he tried to force this awareness out of his consciousness, it was still there, still a powerful wish. But I have worked with dreams enough to know that, if you give them the benefit of the doubt, if you assume they have deeper meaning, that assumption will be rewarded. Besides, why did Manny need a message from the unconscious to tell him something that was true of every person in that program?

What was startling in Manny's dream was the magical quality of the whiskey. While obviously not true of the actual drug alcohol itself, the magicalness conveyed something important about Manny's atti-tude toward alcohol. To him it was not whiskey pure and simple, but the fountain of life, a magical elixir, healing waters. The real drink he needed was from the water of life.

Perhaps an exploration of his dream would have led to an investi-gation of the magical expectations Manny held about alcohol, compar-ing these to the simple, sober reality. Perhaps it would have led to a discussion about where the healing waters that bubbled up in his dream might be found inside rather than outside himself—how he might connect to his inner spiritual resources for healing. Since I didn't see Manny much after that, I will never know for sure.

The Beautiful World of Dreams

When we become aware of dreams, we open the door to a beautiful world, a world full of guidance and wisdom. The unconscious, which speaks to us in dreams, sees things very differently than our conscious ways of seeing. It reminds us of whatever we have been neglecting, thereby pushing us to be more whole and complete, less one-sided. Manny's dream may have been trying to tell him about some positive aspect of drinking. It may have been telling him not only that he had to deal with urges and make them conscious, but that something was missing, that he needed to connect to the font of deeper meanings and wisdom and grace if he were to find healing for the horrible addiction that had so cramped and distorted his life.

People who live in other, less "developed" cultures are sometimes happier than we are, for all our advantages. While there may be far more struggle just to survive, they often lack the neurotic split so common in our own world. Even while they struggle materially, struggle itself is not felt as something alien, but is connected by a web of meaning and faith. We on the other hand, while having far more, have lost this thread of meaning. We have lost our sense of the spiritual. Dreams are a way to heal this split, to reconnect with spiritual meaning.

In therapy, people often try to use reason to figure out what they should do with their lives. Should I marry this person? End this relationship? Should I take this career path? Reason gives some guidance in these matters. But, for the most part, such questions must be answered at a level both higher and deeper than the realm of reason. Intellect and reason are good tools for helping us figure out how to get what we want. But they are poor tools for discovering what we want in the first place. Reason alone cannot tell you whether you should be a salesperson or a stockbroker, an athlete or a software programmer. But once the heart knows what it wants, reason can help you get there.

I recall a childhood friend who told me that his parents gave him three choices: he could be anything he wanted so long as it was a doctor, a lawyer, or an accountant. My friend became a doctor. Years later, when asked if he was happy doing what he did, he could only shrug his shoulders and say, "It's what I do."

From the ego point of view, from the point of view of small self, his parents' advice was wise. Those of us who grew up in the 1960s have learned some difficult lessons about neglecting the part of life that is concerned with making our way in the world and earning a living. Some of us have struggled terribly in this area. But I wonder if my friend would have been happier if he had followed a different path. What would have happened with him if he had listened within to see where the unconscious—the heart—wanted to lead him? Perhaps he would not have earned such a good living. He might have had difficulties finding his way in that respect. But would he have been happier? Would he have known greater peace? The world cannot afford doctors who have no real passion to help and heal, or who, if they had it once, lost it a long time ago. We would be no worse off if these people had chosen something else to do to earn a living. And they themselves might be happier.

Dreams open us to the heart. They connect us with the spiritual and prevent us from choosing a path that, for all the great practical validity it may have, is sterile and flat, devoid of meaning and joy. Dreams challenge the one-dimensional, narrow view of the small self. It isn't that one point of view is always superior. It isn't that the point of view of the ego, with its practical bent, is always wrong, while the spiritual point of view, with its loftier intentions and designs, is always right. Sometimes we may need to follow more the one, sometimes more the other. But it is vitally important that these two aspects be in communication, establishing harmony and balance.

The Other Side

In the third book of C. S. Lewis's Narnia chronicles, *The Voyage of the Dawn Treader*, the characters are on a long sea voyage. At one point, they come to a dark, misty island. Picking up a swimmer from the sea who is desperately trying to get off the island, they learn it is the island where dreams come true. At first, the crew are ecstatic, taking this to mean that it is a place where wishes and fantasies are fulfilled. They engage in fantasies of meeting long-lost loves and enjoying fabulous wealth and ease. But then they get it: it is the place *where dreams come true*. Not hopes. Not wishes. But where all the terrible, nonsensical things that can happen in a dream happen in waking life. The characters in the book turn and row away from the island with all their might.

Lewis's insight is correct. This is the other side. While the dream-world can bring us a wealth of insight and healing, it is also a difficult, dangerous, and confusing place. It is a place where we are chased by vicious animals and evil demons. It is a place where we are found naked in public, where we do things we would never dream of doing, where we are tested and found wanting, where we experience ourselves as drooling idiots or amoral villains. It is the world of fairy tales, which is not only full of handsome princes and beautiful princesses, but also monsters and goblins and dark dangers.

The reason there are such terrors is not hard to seek. The first things that surface as we begin to work with dreams are the things we deny. If we are overly rational in our approach to life, we are confronted with the irrational, or at least, the nonrational. If we deny our fears, in dreams we are forced to confront them directly. If we view ourselves as good people with no dark side whatsoever, we encounter our unowned evil in this dark watery realm. Whatever we have disowned, whatever we deny as difficult or dangerous, whatever we have trouble seeing because it conflicts with our overly positive view of ourselves—these very things are deposited in the unconscious. And just as in so many stories and legends and fairy tales, if we are to get to the treasure, we must accept the hazards of the journey. We must be willing first to confront the monster.

Every dream works toward wholeness, balance, and well-being. But the process is not always pleasant. We will not always like the messages that come to us. For the path to wholeness lies *through*, not around, the very difficulties we would deny and discount. These darker aspects must be confronted if they are to be healed.

Confronting Ourselves

When Luke Skywalker confronts Darth Vader as the embodiment of the dark side of the Force, the Darth Vader of this encounter is of course an aspect of the hero himself more than an external villain. This is what it means when we eventually learn that indeed Darth

Vader was Luke's own father. For the darkness we confront on the way to wholeness is the darkness within ourselves.

In his book *Healing and Wholeness* (1977), Jungian analyst John Sanford relates the story of a Nazi pilot who was grounded because of a sudden loss of color vision. The symptom was itself symbolic; he saw the world in black and white. He had absolute faith in Hitler and the Nazi movement. He had great admiration for his older brother in his SS uniform, stationed in a death camp. His sister, on the other hand, had joined the resistance. The pilot viewed her as the embodiment of evil. Sent to a Jungian analyst trapped in Berlin by the war, the aviator related dreams in which both his brother and Hitler had black faces, while his sister's face was shining white. Not understanding the message, he could only say that the dreamworld was crazy and backward, where black becomes white and white becomes black—the opposite of his conscious attitude. After visiting his SS brother at a death camp, and seeing firsthand what was going on there, the meaning of the dream gradually became apparent.

For this young pilot, the intrusions of the unconscious were unwelcome and distressing—first with the unwelcome symptom of losing color vision, then with the dream material. They challenged his comfortable, narrow, black-and-white view. But we can easily see from our perspective that the unconscious was attempting to give him important information, however disconcerting. Dream information is always important, and it always aims at our healing. But the more out of balance we are, the more incomplete and distorted our point of view, the more disconcerting the dream material will be.

The Wounded Healer

Throughout the myths, legends, and spiritual traditions of the world we encounter the motif of the wounded healer. American Indian medicine men and other native healers often suffer an illness or initiatory wound early in life. Black Elk, for example, became very ill as a boy. Until he cooperated with and understood the call of the spirit realm—what we might call the unconscious from a psychological perspective—he remained ill. When he stopped resisting, he had a great, elaborate vision, and became able to guide his people through a difficult historical transition.

In the myth of Parsifal, the Fisher King suffers an unhealable wound, but this wound is itself a source of healing. He obviously parallels the sufferings of Christ, who brings healing to a broken world through his own suffering. Again and again, we see this motif that it is the wounded one who brings healing.

In his book *The Wounded Healer* (1972), Catholic priest Henri Nouwen recounts this story from the Talmud:

> Rabbi Yoshua ben Levi came upon Elijah the prophet while he was standing at the entrance of Rabbi Simeron ben Yohai's cave. . . . He asked Elijah, "When will the Messiah come?" Elijah replied,
> "Go and ask him yourself."
> "Where is he?"
> "Sitting at the gates of the city."
> "How shall I know him?"
> "He is sitting among the poor covered with wounds. The others unbind all their wounds at the same time and then bind them up again. But he unbinds one at a time and binds it up again, saying to himself, 'Perhaps I shall be needed: if so I must always be ready so as not to delay for a moment.'"

Here, too, the one who heals is the one who is wounded, who must always be ready should he be called upon to help.

Some of our illnesses and life problems can be seen in part as initiatory events—wounds that call us from a more limited point of view to a more complete one. And perhaps all psychological wounds carry some of this function. Addiction can be just such a wound, particularly if you find yourself increasingly drawn out of your woundedness into the spiritual dimension.

Extend Mindfulness into the Area of Sleep

The key that unlocks the door to dream work is to approach this realm with deep respect. You must know there is great power here, power that can heal, but also power that can wound. You do not enter the temple of Asklepios uninvited. You do not enter it irreverently, or out of mere curiosity. You enter with hushed voice and quiet step. You remove the shoes from your feet, knowing you are entering the realm of the holy.

To approach the temple of dreams as though trying to solve a puzzle is to profane it. While dreams will provide insight, and you will have some experiences of "Aha! I understand!" you must be patient and not too goal oriented. The phrase "dream interpretation" is a little misleading, if taken to mean that you are trying to decode a dream—this means this, and that means that. While insight of that kind can come, it is not the main business of dream work.

The main point of working with dreams is to extend the realm of your awareness, to extend mindfulness into the area of sleep. Just as when you are practicing mindfulness in daily life, you do not ask so much, "What is the meaning of this flower, this sunset, this traffic jam?" but you open to these phenomena with calm awareness. So with dream work. Not all the wisdom from dreams will be translatable into conscious words and meanings. But by the simple act of bringing awareness to dreams, you are already moving toward wholeness.

Sometimes dream work in therapy brings wonderful verbal and intellectual insights. But this is not always so. Nor does it seem to matter a great deal whether such insights come. Just as often, the healing comes from attending to the dream images themselves, by simply working with them, entertaining them in conscious awareness for a time. People often find relief for an oppressive mood or feeling just by doing this, whether or not they have much conscious understanding of the dream material. So while it is good to get whatever conscious insight you can from dream material, don't press too hard. When you do so, you can become desperate to squeeze insight out of the dream material. Dream material resists being squeezed into the narrow mold of our conscious thoughts and interpretations. A process approach is the best way; just be aware of the dream material, work with it, let it penetrate you deeply, and penetrate it with gentle mindfulness. Never try to force or impose a meaning. If meanings come, that is good. If they don't, that is good also.

Exegesis versus Eisegesis

Theology differentiates two modes of scriptural interpretation. *Exegesis* means taking from the text the meaning that is actually there; *eisegesis* means reading into the text whatever you want to see in it. The conclusions you reach regarding the meaning of a passage with these two approaches are dramatically different. Exegesis means listening deeply to the passage, seeing what it is aiming at rather than import your own prejudices and beliefs into it. It means listening to the scripture and letting it speak.

Practice exegesis rather than eisegesis with dream material. *Let the dream speak*. Carl Jung asked his clients repeatedly, "What does the *dream* say?" coming back again and again to the dream itself rather than get too far removed from it in speculations about its meaning.

Working with Dreams

Dream material is elusive and difficult to catch in conscious awareness. For this reason, we need a container. One client I worked with on dreams had a difficult time remembering them. When he started to remember dreams at least occasionally, he said it was as though there were a movie or a television program going on in the corner of his consciousness. He had to learn to pay attention to this process and recognize it as dreaming.

If you have trouble remembering dreams, it helps first to spend the evening quietly before you go to sleep. Try not to fill the time with television, Nintendo, videos, loud music, or the like. Try to avoid too many flashing images or other kinds of disturbances. Give yourself a quiet time—as we all should anyway. Practice walking and sitting meditation, or listening to restful music, or doing some quiet reading.

Second, as you are falling asleep, take a few conscious breaths, and form the intention to allow yourself to remember your dreams. Take the ritual action of setting pen and paper beside your bed. This is a powerful communication to the unconscious that you are ready to listen. Often, this will be enough to help you remember your dreams.

The first step, then, to working with dreams is to begin to remember and record the dream material. As an alternative to writing, tell the dream to a trusted friend. Sometimes this process of telling or recording a dream will already provide some insight into a dream. But remember that respecting this material with your attention is already useful and important, even if you have no idea what it means.

Other Things to Do with a Dream

Beyond the steps of recording a dream or sharing it with a trusted person, here are some other things you can do to integrate these important epistles from the unconscious.

Meditate on the Dream

Breathe in and out, and be present to the atmosphere and content of the dream. Let it penetrate you. Let it speak to you, in its own language, in its own time. Do this for at least five or ten minutes. Since the goal is to establish communication between the conscious and unconscious mind, this is a valuable practice in itself. *Trust the process.*

Associate to the Dream

Take each element of the dream—each character, each object, each event, the location of the dream—and associate to it. For example, if you have a dream in which the family car from your childhood appears, ask yourself what this is, and write down your associations. What comes up for you when you think of that old car?

It is important in doing this that you keep coming back to the dream element itself, rather than associate to your associations. That is, ask yourself, "What comes to my mind about this? What is a car, anyway? What especially is this car, since it was not some car in general but a specific one that occurred to me?" Write down what comes up for you. Keep returning to the car. If the car makes you think of something that happened when you were six, that may be a useful association; but do not go on to ask what *that* incident makes you think of. You might get some interesting connections if you continue to free-associate to each thing that comes up, but it may have nothing to do with the dream. Keep coming back to the dream elements themselves.

Sometimes people try too hard, and interfere with the process of association. Learn to be hands-off. If, while thinking of the car, you find yourself thinking about a friend you used to know, even though you see no obvious connection between the car and this friend, that is a valid association.

It can take a little practice for some people to learn how to do this. Trust that what comes up while you are thinking about a particular dream element is important and in some way related, even if you cannot see a logical relationship.

Associate to each element in the dream until you have several associations. How do you know which association is best? When you get a feeling of "aha!" about some association, trust it. This feeling of "aha!" is often accompanied by a slight physical shift in the feelings in your body, or perhaps by a deep breath or a sigh. Learn to pay attention to these physical sensations. They are telling you that you are on to something important.

Details, Details

Sometimes the most important clues regarding a dream's meaning are embedded in tiny details you might pass by in telling or writing the dream. Make sure you pay attention to things like the environment in which the dream takes place, and who the people are around you. For example, you might dream of a friend of yours, but in the dream your brown-haired friend has blonde hair. Pay attention to this. Ask yourself whose hair this blonde hair is like. Your dream may have condensed several people into one, perhaps indicating that it is not the specific individual who is important, but whatever these people have in common.

"If It Were My Dream . . ."

If you are finding it difficult to free-associate, you can enlist the help of a trusted person to play "if it were my dream." Tell the person your dream, and ask him what comes to mind when he thinks of the particular dream elements you are stuck on. If you had a dream of swimming in the ocean, for example, and you cannot imagine what this means, you might ask someone what comes to mind when he thinks of swimming in the ocean. Get several associations from him, and see if you respond to any of them with that internal "aha!" Sometimes someone else will have an association that feels right, or at least that makes you think of something that fits better than what you had gotten so far.

To play this game effectively, you need to protect the creative atmosphere of your play. If you reject everything other people offer, they tend to stop having ideas. Instead, just listen to what the other person says, take it in, and see how it feels to you. Then just say something like, "Uh-huh. What else?" And continue. If something she offers does strike a chord, of course, talk about this. But do not offer negative feedback.

It is important to remember, especially in playing this game, that *the dreamer is always the ultimate arbiter of what a dream means*. This is so, even if the person who is assisting you is an expert dream interpreter such as a therapist. This is especially true when the dream element you are associating to has an obvious personal dimension, such as in the case of the old family car. You are more likely to know the meaning of such a personal historical symbol than anyone else.

Active Imagination

Sometimes a dream has an unfinished quality. For instance, you might dream that you are being chased by something, and wake up in the midst of the chase. Obviously, such a dream has not reached a conclusion of any kind. With such a dream, you can take out your journal, sit before it quietly, taking a few conscious breaths to calm and center yourself, and then let yourself enter the atmosphere of the dream. Imagine the dream unfolding, letting it develop any way it seems to want to go, not trying to make it come to any particular kind of ending. Watch what happens as though you were watching a movie, just letting it unfold, and record it in your dream journal.

Similarly, you may meet characters in your dream who seem important in some way. Sometimes, for example, we meet people from our past whom we have not thought of in years. And sometimes, too, we meet characters in a dream who have an obviously numinous, magical quality. It is very helpful at times to let a dialogue unfold in your imagination between you as your conscious self or ego and such dream figures. Ask this person a question. Then let him respond. Write down whatever you hear.

This technique, which Carl Jung called *active imagination*, may be the single most important thing you can do with your dream. The insights that come to us from dreams are not always of a rational nature. You may not be able to articulate them or put them into words that make sense. Such nonrational insights come from the deeper, older parts of the brain, which does not think in words but in potent symbols. Even when you are able to put some insights from a dream into words, it is always a mistake to assume that you have completely captured the dream's meaning. The communication between the unconscious mind and the conscious mind is a little like someone who speaks Chinese but no English trying to communicate with someone who speaks English but no Chinese. The language each uses is built on such a different foundation that it is difficult going for each to understand the other. If the two individuals work hard at it, making full use of gestures, facial expressions, and so forth, they may develop a rough idea of what the other one is trying to say. Even so—even if they each come up with a rough translation of what the other person is saying—they will still miss a lot of the nuance and subtlety of the other's message. They may even miss the point altogether. It would certainly be a mistake to assume that one's translation into one's own language was a valid and complete interpretation.

The difference between the language of the conscious mind and that of the unconscious mind is much greater, however, than the difference between English and Chinese. For however different these languages are, they are both products of the rational, conscious mind. This is not the case with the conscious and the unconscious.

Thus it is important to remember that no formula of words will ever be completely adequate for capturing the meaning of a dream. Fortunately, understanding a dream at this level, while helpful, is not critical. What is really most important is to bring these aspects of self—conscious and unconscious as we call them, for lack of better terms—into *relationship* with each other. Active imagination does this supremely well.

Sometimes people resist this process. They object: "But I just made it all up." And this is true of course. But ask yourself another question: Where did you make it up from? For after all, you also in a sense made up your dream to begin with.

Dream Language Is Symbolic

A woman dreamed that she was in a swimming pool with her young daughter on her back. She was okay for a while, but as time went on, she was becoming exhausted. The weight of the child was pushing her under water, and she could not get air. Her husband, meanwhile, was trying to take a picture of mother and child swimming together, but the camera was not working.

While to fully interpret such a dream one would need the personal associations and involvement of the dreamer, it is not hard to make some guesses about what it means. This woman is drowning under the weight of child rearing, while her husband does not seem to "get the picture." There may be other meanings. The child, for example, may stand for something else, especially if it is not her own child. The child may stand for a project or endeavor that is about the same age as the dream figure. But it would be unlikely to think that this dream was literally about swimming or photography.

A man who was about to begin a career as a public speaker had a dream in which he was playing in a rock band, but his amplifier was too small. This individual had played in a band in his younger days. The unconscious borrowed this experience to symbolize his present endeavor as a speaker. The too small amplifier meant there was insufficient power to get his message out to the public. He needed a more powerful means to broadcast his message than had so far been available to him. Again, exploring personal associations would be important. Why did the dream specifically use his rock band experience instead of something else? Do the shape and size of the amplifier tell us anything? The general thrust of the dream message in this case was relatively clear, but one never reaches a point where one has completely and fully explicated a symbol like the small amplifier. It is a little like what singer Bob Dylan reportedly said when asked what one of his songs meant. Dylan said that if he could have expressed it another way, he would have. Dreams likewise try to communicate with us as directly as possible. But the language they speak is the language of symbols. And a symbol can never be reduced to a verbal formula.

It is important to remember that dreams speak a special language, a language of symbols. Symbols are not signs that stand interchangeably for something else. The meaning of a symbol can never completely be put into words. In the Buddhist saying that the teaching of the Buddha is a finger pointing at the moon, the word *moon* is a symbol. Perhaps we could even offer that it means something like "enlightenment." But the symbol itself is richer than that. And besides, saying the moon is a symbol for *enlightenment* only substitutes one symbol for another. Those of us who are not yet enlightened do not really know what enlightenment is any more than we know what the symbol of the moon means. So it is very important to keep an open mind toward the meaning of dream symbols and never feel that you have fully explicated the meaning of a dream or a dream symbol.

Symbols must not be confused with signs. A sign simply stands for something else, meaning no more and no less than that other thing. If we interpreted the amplifier to stand for a new speaking contract, this would be to see it as a sign. But as a symbol, it can have many dimensions. It might mean the new contract, but also the personal power of the speaker to project a certain quality, and many other things as well. Treat dream material as symbols, not signs.

Having said that, however, there are nonetheless some regularities to dream symbolism. Water, for example, often stands for the unconscious; a house may stand for the psyche itself. Symbol dictionaries can sometimes give you some clues about symbols, though they also may confuse you more often than not. But since the nature of symbols is never fully explicable, it should already be apparent to you that it is not very helpful to use a book of dream symbols (different from a book of symbols per se), especially those which say baldly that this means that or x means y. This reduces the symbol to a mere sign, one thing standing in for another.

You will therefore want to avoid dream interpretations that seem a little too neat or pat, and remember that it is the process of working with this material that is most important, not being able to specify exactly what a dream means.

Controlling the Flow

Since dreams have the built-in safety valve of letting you forget any material that is too threatening for you to integrate, reducing the flow of dream material is rarely a problem. But occasionally, people get overwhelmed by unconscious material. If you find that working with dream material has been leaving you a bit depressed, or anxious, or haunted by the dream material in a disturbing way for hours after waking, this may be an indication that it is too much too soon. You may need to reduce the flow of material from the unconscious toward conscious awareness to a level that you can integrate more easily.

Since the problem with most of us today is one of learning to remember dreams at all rather than remember them too much, it is generally easy to reduce the flow of dream material. All you need do is go back to what you were doing before you began working with dreams. Stop recording them for a while. Cease all effort to try to hold on to dreams by mentally rehearsing them or telling anyone about them. Then when you feel ready to listen in to your unconscious again, at first just pay attention to dream material that feels particularly powerful or important in some way. This will generally be enough to prevent you from continuing to get overwhelmed. If it is not, this may be because there is some urgency for you in integrating this material. You may have been cut off for too long from some important aspects of who you are. In this case, you might like to find a therapist to work with who is skilled at dream work.

Of course, if you are already engaged in a therapeutic process involving dreams, there is already increased safety for you because of the therapeutic alliance. In this case, it may not be necessary to turn the flow down even if the dream material is quite disturbing, though you can talk about this possibility with your therapist.

The Result of Work with Dreams

Sometimes there is immediate relief from working with a dream. Since the purpose of a dream is to correct imbalance, this can happen at times by the simple act of remembering a dream, even if you don't understand its meaning or have not done much work with it. Somewhat more frequently, a feeling of relief comes from working with a dream. You may feel subtle or even not so subtle shifts in your body tension or changes in mood states after working a dream through, giving it your most accepting, positive, mindful energy.

Nonetheless, you should not be surprised if you do not feel any immediate results from working with a dream. Sometimes, even after your best efforts to work with a dream, you still may not have much conscious awareness of what the dream is trying to communicate. But if you pay attention over weeks and months, you may notice an increased sense of wholeness and well-being emerge out of your dream work. You may find that you are less prone to negative mood states and that they linger for a shorter period of time when they do emerge. You may experience renewed energy, both physically and mentally. Look for these changes. They can only help you stay on track with your recovery process. But since people are geared more toward noticing what is wrong than what is right, you may not catch these gradual changes unless you pay attention.

Research on changing addictive behavior supports a process orientation toward change. As discussed earlier, people go through specifiable changes, in general cycling through the stages of change several times before leaving it behind. Even when you examine stories of what seem, on the surface, to be sudden and dramatic changes—when people report that one day they just gave it all over to God and quit struggling—a closer examination reveals that there were many preparatory events and subtle changes that led up to this point. Outwardly, the change may appear sudden and dramatic; but inwardly, there were subtle, cumulative changes occurring that eventually added up to the large change on the exterior level.

As with meditating, mindfulness in daily life, journaling, and all the practices recommended in this book, so it is also with dreaming. The most important thing is to have faith in the process, to cultivate an inner knowing that positive changes are occurring day by day, though they may be too subtle for you to notice all at once.

Nowhere is trusting the process more important than in working with dreams. In a certain sense, the more disturbing the dream material, the more healing it may ultimately be. That which disturbs the most will have the greatest healing effect when you can shine the light of awareness on it and integrate it. Impatience is one of the greatest obstacles to change and growth. Hidden beneath the surface, seeds are sprouting, sending roots deep into the earth. But if in our impatience, we pull them out to check how they are doing, no growth will be possible.

You can do it. The work of mindfulness is always about accepting how we are and how life is right now, not about trying to earn worthiness for some future achievement of inhuman perfection. Respect and accept the messages dreams give you as a way of accepting yourself just as you are right now. Dangerous people are not the ones who know their own darkness and shadow side, but those who do not. Dreams can help you be aware of all that you are, good and bad alike.

Doorway Eight
WORKING

It isn't enough that we have meaningful work. What is required is work that satisfies the soul.

—Thomas Moore,
The Re-Enchantment of Everyday Life (1996)

∽ॐ∾

Practice mindfulness at work. A mindful life involves mindfulness in all areas of life. Practicing mindfulness at work can help you stay calm and centered there as well.

∽ॐ∾

A Fork in the Road: Amanda's Story

Arriving home from work, Amanda felt tired and empty. It was as if she needed compensation for what she had been enduring all day long. If she put the feeling into words, it would be something like "I've worked hard all day, now where's my reward?" Her immediate answer was a glass of wine.

While Amanda would not qualify for a formal diagnosis of alcohol dependence, lately she had become concerned about her drinking. There were too many nights spent alone, too many empty wine bottles around. Increasingly she felt she needed wine to cope. After attending one of our mindfulness workshops, she had begun to practice. The first fruit of her increased awareness was the knowledge that what she was doing wasn't working. She saw clearly that instead of restoring her spirits and giving her a reward, lately her wine drinking left her depleted, tired, and sad.

Amanda sensed she was at a fork in the road. Would she continue the destructive pattern, or do something else? She considered practicing sitting or walking meditation. But her thoughts kept swinging back and forth between nurturing herself in this way, or drinking. If too many more nights go by with her choosing the wine, she might well be on her way to a serious alcohol problem.

Work as Foundation

Amanda's job is not awful. She is well paid and has great benefits, and in the limited Albuquerque job market, she feels lucky to have her job. But there is a subtle feeling of constriction from it. It is like wearing shoes that are just a little too tight. You put them on, at first aware that they pinch a little, but then forget about them and go about your day. Only when you take them off at the end of the day and feel the relief do you realize how tight they were and how much they were binding your feet.

Unless you are independently wealthy, chances are you have to work. The stay-at-home spouse is becoming a rarity. Now virtually everyone, male or female, has to work just to get by. The majority of us are just barely doing so. If you work full-time, more than one-third of your waking hours are spent at work, and many of the remaining hours are spent preparing for work or recovering from it. If you work forty hours a week for forty years, with perhaps two weeks of vacation, that totals eighty thousand hours of this precious, limited human life—the life that the Buddha described as but a flash of lightning. And even more important than the time, work requires the majority of our energy and attention, little of which remains for the rest of life.

We often say that work is not the most important thing to us. We say family is more important, our relationships are more important, our spirituality is more important, our friendships are more important. But when you consider how much of your time and energy are spent on those things relative to time and energy spent working, it does not add up. Either what we say is not true, and work is really what is most important, or else we are living out of harmony with ourselves and with what really matters.

Psychologist Abraham Maslow introduced the concept of a hierarchy of human needs. Before we can take care of upper-level needs like self-actualization and creativity, we must first have established a secure base at the lower levels. In other words, we must meet basic needs for food, clothing, and shelter before we can give much attention to aesthetics or personal growth.

It may be a little more complicated than this, but nonetheless, most of us must give attention and energy to our day-to-day survival, meeting basic human needs for ourselves and those who depend on us. And for most of us, no matter how deep our spiritual side, work is a necessity.

Work as Curse

The Creation story in the second chapter of Genesis depicts the start of human life in a garden. In the garden, all our needs are met. We live a life of natural ease and grace, needing only to pick our choice of the abundantly available fruits of the earth. However, some sort of human overreaching—depicted as the eating of the forbidden fruit—changes all this forever. Whatever this transgression was (the Bible gives no indication it was about sex), we currently find ourselves banished, forever shut out of the garden. And as a consequence, we now must work to live.

> Because you . . . have eaten of the tree of which I commanded you, "You shall not eat of it," cursed is the ground because of you; in toil you shall eat of it all the days of your life. . . . In the sweat of your face you shall eat bread till you return to the ground. (Genesis 3:17–19)

This is certainly a dark view of work. But even if you do not subscribe to a biblical point of view, it remains a foundational story, one which has penetrated the consciousness of Western society deeply.

But if people in the agrarian society of ancient Israel could take such a negative view of their work, our present-day situation is even more serious, and far more deeply alienated. Most of us no longer work on our own land, with our own families around to help, raising crops that will primarily feed ourselves. At least when people did so, work was of a piece with the rest of life, not some separate corner, some strange and alien thing done solely as a means. Growing crops and milking cows were just what you did, and it made sense in an immediate kind of way. Compare this, for example, to buying and selling commodity futures on the market. This is not only a more stressful way to earn a living (since the trader is trying to predict future events), but it is also several layers of abstraction removed from the tangible task of growing produce which the trader, her family, and perhaps a few neighbors will eat. In other words, it is a far more alienated way of earning your bread.

If the author of Genesis was aware of this difficulty about work, what would he think of the conditions under which so many of us work today? Not only are we working for intangible results that do not directly feed and nourish us, but so many of us are underappreciated, humiliated, treated like children incapable of taking our own initiative or bringing a task to completion without managers breathing down our necks, continually pressured to produce more with less, robbed of the credit we deserve for our efforts, and surrounded with difficult people on top of everything else. No wonder even a not particularly unusual or stressful workday can trigger episodes of abuse and excess.

Work as Blessing

Being more aware includes awareness of the stories that continue to shape our perceptions and beliefs. For not only does the Genesis view of work capture an important truth, but this truth also continues to operate in the Western psyche, shaping our perceptions of and relationship to work. Many of us have unconsciously accepted the situation in Genesis, seeing ourselves as doomed to perform empty, difficult tasks all day long, using the best of our time and energy on things with no intrinsic meaning. It is indeed as though we are under a divine curse, laboring like galley slaves to fulfill someone else's purposes, all so we can just survive, maybe enjoying weekends and all too fleeting holidays and vacations, hanging on by our fingernails for twenty or thirty years until we retire. This is a Faustian pact, a selling of our souls to the demon of security, who often reneges on the deal anyway when the company we've worked for decides to "downsize"—a terrible modern euphemism for leaving people out of work.

But this is by no means the whole story about work. Even some of the most "meaningless" jobs have blessing aspects as well as curse aspects. If you yourself have ever been unemployed—or as we are more likely to say about ourselves, "between jobs"—you know the terror of this situation. Such periods teach the value of work, even in some of its emptier forms. It is difficult for many of us to feel good about ourselves when others are going off to work, and we are facing another day with little structure and less certainty. And while some jobs damage our self-esteem, nothing is more damaging to self-esteem than being unable to pay bills and meet material needs.

Chinese Zen master Hyakujo performed hard physical labor alongside his students into his eighties. His students, being concerned about him, but also knowing that he would not listen to their advice, decided to hide his tools. Their plan backfired, however. Hyakujo did not work, but he also did not eat. This went on for several days before his anxious students decided to put his tools back. When he could work again, the master started eating again as well. His one comment: "No work, no food."

Even in Zen, which emphasizes being rather than doing, food and work cannot ultimately be separated. Food simply tastes better when we have worked for it. There is nothing more debilitating for a human being than feeling useless. That is why nursing home residents become stronger and more alert when given responsibility for the care of a plant or a pet. They have something to do, something that depends upon them, and they rise to the occasion.

If we are to be truly aware and mindful at work, this important aspect of life, it is vital that we be aware not only of the curse aspects of work, but also of its blessing aspects. Both aspects deserve awareness. If the curse continues to operate in an unconscious way, we will not even know we are making a choice when we decide to stay in a job we dislike because we view it as our fate. But if we are unaware of the blessing dimension of our employment, we may cut ourselves off too quickly from the foundational level of our needs hierarchy, perhaps quitting on the spot some uncomfortable job, but leaving ourselves unprotected in a cold world.

It is cheap and easy to say, "Leave the rat race, drop out, quit, try something you really love." This countercultural message may at times be the right thing to do, but unless it is a conscious choice— unless it is done with full awareness of the costs of cutting yourself off from the blessing aspect of work—and unless this choice is made with full awareness of who you are and what you need to feel comfortable, including your own tolerance for risk and need for security, the liberating drama of quitting may backfire. You may suffer a lot. Decisions about work must be made with deep mindfulness, with honest acceptance of who you really are and what you really need.

On the other side, however, is another truth: people who have found their way to work they love, and work that also meets their material needs with some level of abundance, have often been people who were willing to take some risks, willing to leave the beaten path for the road less traveled. Often such life stories include many early failures before finding the right niche. Such people have often tried this business or that profession or this line of work, failing repeatedly before reaching success. The rest of us may envy them, but want no part of the early trial-and-error process.

PRACTICE

Meditate on Work as Blessing and Curse

Spend five or ten minutes or a full meditation period contemplating work, this important area of your life. Just let the whole experience of work turn over and over in your mind as you breathe in and out, without particularly trying to grasp at anything. Turn these questions over in your mind, not forcing an answer: In what ways are you operating our of the idea of work as curse? What aspects of your work fit in with this, causing you to feel heavy and burdened? In what ways is your work a blessing? What aspects feel light and enjoyable? Consider not just external factors like earning money, but intrinsic aspects of your experience at work as well. How can you capitalize on positive aspects and decrease negative aspects?

When you are done meditating, record your insights on paper. Read them over slowly, breathing in and out, taking in what you have written, trusting your Buddha nature, your insight.

The Watercourse Way

Consider the way of water as it floods an open field. It extends a thin finger this way, going as far as it can go by virtue of its own center of gravity and the contours of the land, then perhaps moving in another direction altogether, always seeking its own level, trying something, then trying something else, never attached to one particular way. This Taoist metaphor teaches a fundamental aspect of how to live, and applies quite nicely to a fruitful work life as well. To allow yourself to flow in a new direction if there seems no way to proceed on the present path, then perhaps changing again, and yet again, can indeed be the way of wisdom. Some particular course may "work," allowing you to reach the ultimate goal of the sea. But if you understand the way of water, it is not really so important whether this happens—whether you are successful by any external standard. What matters is the willingness to flow, to follow your own nature.

Beverly had a job where she was loved and respected, but felt an inner call to move on. For a long time she tried to ignore it. Even when she had secretly decided, she did not let her left hand know what her right hand was doing, acting as though no final decision had been made. But it had. Packing all her belongings into her Toyota, she made her way across country, circling around in the Southwest before finally settling in Albuquerque. There she and I met, and Beverly started a new life. Not all aspects of her journey were smooth or easy. But it had become unthinkable for her to stay, despite the risks. You hold in your hands one result of her decision.

I have always felt a desire to be a spiritual leader, and becoming a pastor seemed the natural way to do it. Yet there was a deep incompatibility between me and the pastoral role. I kept wanting to believe I was just not at the right church, but after serving in several churches, I had to conclude this was not the problem. I just did not fit well into the church setting. Eventually, slowly, it became clear it was time to leave. Since I had enjoyed counseling and felt I might have some talent for it, I decided to pursue a doctorate in psychology. It was a difficult, sometimes frightening experience. Nor was my entrance into the psychological profession smooth and easy, since economic changes had hit the field hard. But the call to move on was irresistible. I had to follow it.

Were these the right choices? It would depend a lot on your perspective. But for both of us, as for most people who venture from the secure path, there was a compelling inner call that could not be ignored.

Work and Slips

If your work has little to feed and free your spirit, then no matter what the financial rewards, it is causing suffering in you. It is not just a matter of whether things are terrible. Often a lot of pain hides behind innocuous phrases like "It's not so bad, really." Poet Robert Bly said that if you are not being admired, you are being hurt. If you are capable, and if you invest good energy into your work, *you have the right to be admired and appreciated for what you do*. If that is not happening where you work, it is important to let yourself be mindful of your pain. Though it may feel better in the short run to deny it, it is only by honestly experiencing your pain that you will find the motivation to look for other possibilities.

A lot of the vague emptiness experienced at the end of the day may be of this variety—the "oh, it's not that bad" kind of feeling. But of course, sometimes it really is that bad. Sometimes it is more than a matter of being unappreciated, it is one of being actively abused, scolded, belittled, or humiliated. It is little wonder that people who work in such jobs are tempted to relapse at the end of the workday. Here the practice of mindfulness can center you, helping you heal and transform your pain, helping you to know when, no matter how frightening it may seem, it is time to make a change, giving you the strength to be aware of this and do it in a reasonable, planned way that reduces the risk.

PRACTICE

Find Alternative Ways to Restore Yourself after Work

Preventing relapse is more than stopping the addictive behavior. It is also about finding satisfying alternatives, finding other things to do. You need not only to stop following the addictive habit energy, but to do something else instead. Even if you are not in danger of relapse, it is important for your well-being to find ways to restore yourself after work.

On a sheet of paper or in your journal, list as many alternatives to using as you can think of to restore yourself after the workday. To begin with, do this without censoring your ideas, writing down even the ones that seem a little silly or impractical, so as to ensure a creative flow of thought. Try to come up with a lot of ideas—say, twenty or more—for the more you have, the more likely it is that you will have one on the list that you can use when you need to.

When you have made your initial list, place an asterisk by the alternatives that seem the best to you, so you can look at these first. Next time you come home from work a little tired, empty, or sad, take out your list. Choose the one that is the most appealing and put it into practice.

Starting Over

The poor work history of some recovering people adds another dimension to the dilemma of work. If your addiction has been strong enough that you have lost many days of work because of it, or come to work impaired or even just not at your best, it is important to be mindful of the connection between your own behavior and how you are being treated. It is possible that you are not treated well because your own behavior has caused damage to your work situation.

When that is the case, it is important to acknowledge it. It is not a matter of punishing yourself for this, or succumbing to guilt. It is a practical matter of rebuilding broken trust, of reestablishing a record of reliability that inspires confidence. Let your inner voice guide you regarding what you need to do. Is it possible to heal the damage done where you work, to show over time a new attitude that will win over coworkers and employers? Or do you need to move on because so much damage has been done that it feels too onerous to consider trying to repair it? Have you done so much damage to your work life that you need to accept a lower-level position for a while, perhaps to work yourself back up again to the kind of responsibility you had formerly? To some extent, every recovering person is in a phase of *starting over* with regard to her work life. Starting over can be a difficult process. The phrase implies ending and difficulty, but it also implies positive possibilities. It implies new life and new opportunities, opportunities which might never have been open to you otherwise. Mindfulness of the cycle of life on earth teaches that death and rebirth are built into the very nature of things. Sometimes it is time to let go of what was and what might have been, to come back into the present reality, to take in its healing possibilities deeply and work commitedly with what is available here and now. This is the path of healing.

Rebuilding Your Work Life

If you are in a rebuilding phase, it is important to find positive aspects about your work and be mindful of them, even if you know that your present position is a stopgap measure. Practice giving some of your best energy to whatever you may be doing. Practice breathing and smiling. Give of yourself. Do not be someone who just clings to the formalities of a job description, but try to make a positive difference wherever you can. While a supervisor who repeatedly expects you to put in more time than you are supposed to may be unreasonable, it is also unreasonable as an employee to be so much of a clock-watcher that you fail to complete an important task simply because it would have taken a little more time to do than you had in your official workday.

In the Buddhist practice of the Five Remembrances, the fifth remembrance is that our deeds (karma) are our only true possessions. Whatever we practice today generates a momentum that carries over into tomorrow. If we practice being an angry, unhappy person today, we increase our potential to be angry and unhappy in the future. If we practice being an uncaring employee today, this injures us—even if the job we presently have is temporary. By being an uncaring, careless employee today, we run the risk of getting stuck in that way of being and taking it with us even into work that we care about.

So it is important to do your best within a given situation, even when you are not appreciated as much as you should be. Or you may be hurting yourself as much as anyone.

Difficult People

One of the hardest aspects of work is encounters with difficult people. It is hard enough when you encounter difficult people in the general public, as you would in a sales position for example. But at least in such a case, there is some professional distance between you and the other people to insulate you a little from their psychospiritual toxins. You usually do not have to deal with them on a daily basis. But when the difficult individual is someone you must work with regularly and closely, such as a coworker, or worse still, a supervisor or employer, this can put your mindfulness to the test.

The first hurdle to deal with in such cases is psychological: if you are drawn to spiritual practice, you may have an image of yourself as someone who is, or at least should be, continually saintly in demeanor, and whose spiritual depth and power are supposed to change and heal the environment simply by your own depth of mindful presence. And in a certain way, this is true. Your deep presence can exert a healing influence on those around you. However, some interpersonal environments are simply so toxic that it is unreasonable to expect that you will heal them. Far more likely, they will wound you. Even if your mindfulness is deep, some environments are simply overwhelming. Even Christ was unable to work miracles in some situations because of the unbelief of those around him. In other words, even if your mindfulness is quite solid, there are environments that will take you down instead of being elevated by you. And of course, if you are new to mindfulness practice, it is even more unrealistic to expect that you will be able to overcome the poisonous atmosphere found in some workplaces. Ultimately the best strategy may be to leave such workplaces as soon as you can make a reasonable plan to do so.

The Buddha once had a conversation with an effective horse trainer. He asked the trainer how he handled his horses. The trainer explained that some horses respond best to gentleness; others require the whip, and some others, a combination of both. A few even have to be killed for the sake of the stable. The trainer then asked the Buddha how he taught his followers. He said he did it the same way. Some need a lot of gentleness, some do best with strict discipline, and some need a combination of the two. But some needed to be killed. The horse trainer was surprised. How could this peaceful, gentle teacher talk of killing? The Buddha explained that, for the sake of the whole community, it was sometimes necessary to ask a follower to leave the community.

Of course, whichever kind of treatment the Buddha found helpful in the case of a particular student, the Buddha's compassion was behind it. It is no more kind to be lax with those who need strictness than it is to be strict with those who need a lot of gentleness. Even those whom he "killed"—meaning, in this case, forcing them to leave the community—were treated with compassion. A follower who did not uphold the standards of practice of the community would first be engaged in every possible way to try to help him change. But eventually, if despite every effort and despite great patience, such an individual still did not follow the way of practice, he would be asked to leave. In some cases, the Buddha allowed a person back into the community many times after having asked him to leave for being disruptive.

This is a lesson in the flexibility of mindfulness. Mindfulness always leads to compassionate action, but if we are mindful, we are flexible regarding what type of action is truly compassionate, and what type of action only appears to be so. There can be a wide gulf between mere niceness on the one hand, and true, mindful compassion on the other.

Your mindfulness may teach you to continue to act in a patient, outwardly kind manner with some people. With others, however, it may be important to stand up for yourself more, and resist being treated in an abusive manner. And in some situations, you may need to leave the environment of the other person or, if you have the authority, ask her to leave. In other words, you may have to find another job, or fire someone. But all of this can be a form of compassion when mindfulness is present.

Metta Meditation for People at Work

If you are in a work situation that you may be able to help transform and heal, then practicing metta meditation for the people you work with can be very powerful. Metta meditation is a way to train your own mind and cultivate compassion. For the first step in transforming an outward situation is to transform your own awareness.

You may recall from the Doorway on meditation that metta meditation begins with yourself first, which is the starting point of all love and compassion, and then spreads out in concentric circles of increasing difficulty—your most beloved person, your close friends and family, then neutral people, enemies, and finally, all beings. It is possible for you to have coworkers in all these circles. And if the situation is transformable, metta meditation will help a lot.

In the context of work, however, it is important that you not be in a hurry to get through all of the circles or levels. Staying, for example, at the level of self-love may be the most important part of this practice. If you are being abused by a work situation, metta meditation toward yourself may be the most important practice. You should stay at this level for a good while, perhaps many meditation sessions, and only when you feel some deep nurturing and healing occurring for yourself consider going on to other levels. Without a deeply established self-love, it will not be possible to extend loving kindness to those who hurt you. Also, these levels are not really separate anyway. Since in the Buddhist understanding, we are all deeply connected to each other, giving loving kindness to ourselves affects the other people around us as well. The converse is also true: loving our enemies is a form of self-healing.

So if your work presents interpersonal challenges and difficulties, practice metta meditation. But be sure to spend a generous amount of time and energy on yourself before you try to bring loving kindness to those with whom you have difficulty. Take your time. Never feel that you have to cover all of the levels in one sitting if you are not ready.

Dream Work and Work Work

If you have been doing work with dreams, you have another tool that can guide you through difficult work choices and help with difficult relationships. An important aspect of this is *taking back the projection*. When you work with dreams, you come to see that each dream is ultimately about yourself, even if there are other people in the dream from your daily life. From this perspective, each dream character is a part of you. So if you have a dream about someone whom you dislike, who is doing hurtful things, it is important to see that this is not only the other person, but also a part of you. After all, you are the origina-tor of your own dreams. This allows you to take responsibility for your life situation, and by being forgiving and kind to those aspects of your-self which are difficult to accept and deal with, to begin to extend this kindness also to the difficult people around you.

Skill

A popular expression has it that the road to hell is paved with good intentions. Behind this trite phrase lies an important truth: It is not enough to have positive intent. More is required. A mindfulness-based spirituality is very much in tune with this idea. Even if your heart is full of love and compassion, you must learn skillful ways to express these feelings, or else you may do great harm.

When someone at work treats you in an unkind manner, the first thing to do is resolve to breathe and smile. This is not always an easy practice, but it is an immensely important one. By returning to your breathing, you unite body and mind. You return to yourself, to your mindfulness. Only then will you stand a chance of being able to make a response that is helpful, or at least that does not make the situation worse.

So be clear about this in your own mind. You might even like to rehearse it mentally a few times, recalling difficult situations with other people, and visualizing yourself as coming back to your breath and finding your smile. Only then will you be able to respond in accord with some of the suggestions below or in other appropriate ways.

For example, if we are wrongly accused of something, most of us usually catch our breath and breathe shallowly, then defend ourselves or even counterattack. None of these is likely to be the most construc-tive response. If you are mindful, there are other possibilities. More skillful approaches involve both inner and outer strategies.

PRACTICE

Transform Your Thinking

When you are in a difficult situation with another person, use one of the following gathas as you breathe:

"Breathing in and out, I see this person as someone
who just wants to be happy and avoid pain, like me."

"Breathing in and out, I visualize myself and this person as we will both be three hundred years from
now."

"Breathing in and out, the pain I feel is the pain that is
in this other person."

"Breathing in and out, I see myself as a five-year-old
child."

"Breathing in and out, I see this person as a five-year-
old child."

You might like to rehearse these responses mentally, visualizing yourself doing them in difficult situations. Psychological research shows that mental rehearsal increases our chances
of being able to follow through in the actual situation.

Skillful Speech

After you have come back to your breath and reminded yourself of one
of the gathas above, then what?

One of the first things you can do after you calm yourself and breathe
is to use reflection. *Summarize* back to the other person what she is saying, to make sure you really understand it. This is already powerful if
done with calmness and presence. Here the person is angry at you, and
all you show in response is a desire to make sure you understand.

Another approach is to *ask for more information*. The natural tendency toward blame or accusation is a form of defensiveness. But
defensiveness keeps the cycle going. When you act defensively, it con-
vinces the other person that you are indeed guilty, even if this is not
the case at all. Sensing this from you, the other person may continue
to attack. No matter how outrageous the attack or accusation, if you
remain open and calm, and ask the other person to explain what he
means, this will often deflate his anger.

Another strategy is to *agree with part of what the other person is saying*.
For example, if someone has accused you of being controlling, isn't it
true that we all seek to be in control some times? Even if someone says
you are stupid, don't we all act stupidly from time to time? It can derail

a person's anger (and confuse her quite a bit besides) if you admit this, and then perhaps follow up with a request for more information.

Also, *use humor*. Nothing helps us to lighten a heavy situation more than a good laugh. For a tense situation, the best kind of humor is not sarcastic humor, and certainly not humor at the expense of the other person. If the humor is to be at someone's expense, let it be a little bit at your own. If you can breathe and smile and find your calmness, you may be able to touch a seed of laughter within yourself that you can invite the other person to share.

Some situations are so outrageous that it is difficult to hold on to your calmness. But even when it is not possible to make a verbal response that brings some healing to the situation, do your best to hold on to your serenity. At least you will not escalate a bad situation.

One day I received a phone message from someone wanting an appointment to begin therapy. Trying to be responsive to someone in pain, I called him several times over the next few days. A few days later, as I was eating lunch in my office at noontime, this individual showed up, accusing me of everything imaginable, saying I was harassing him with my repeated phone calls. This was very startling. I had never even seen this person before, so at first I did not connect him with the person I'd been calling. To be attacked so suddenly, with no advance warning, was very difficult. Yet I knew this man was in great pain. I could see he was in a paranoid state, possibly psychotic. I could barely imagine his loneliness and fear. My attempts to be welcoming and to reach out to him had been misperceived, and I knew that, given his state of mind, anything I said would be similarly misperceived, and simply taken over into his paranoid fantasies. Breathing in and out, I quietly told him several times, "You need to leave now," until finally, not being able to hook me into more of a discussion, he did just that. I found this very upsetting, and I must admit, I was still a little scattered for my next therapy hour. But by later that afternoon, with the help of a lot of conscious breathing, I was able to calm back down.

Everything Is Best

When we are seeking the spiritual path, we do so because we have begun to see through some of the traps that continue to cause us cycle after cycle of pain. We are looking for a way out, a way to experience peace, joy, and happiness. But there is always a risk of using our spirituality to hide from the world. True spirituality gives us the strength to face life, to be in it fully, to do what is at hand and what needs to be done, taking care of the present moment. It is one of the strengths of the way of mindfulness that it emphasizes this.

Walking one day in the market, a Zen master named Banzan heard a customer ask a butcher for the best piece of meat in his shop. The butcher told him that everything in his shop is the best; there was no piece of meat in his shop that was not the best. At that moment Banzan became enlightened.

When you can adopt the perspective that what comes to you is the best, you can stop worrying about what may come tomorrow, or whether you should have done something other than what you did yesterday, or whether you should be doing what you are doing now. You can be present, and touch the positive elements in your life just as they are. When you can accept that, whatever you might choose to do in the future, today *this* is your work, and *this work* right in front of you is your spiritual practice, you will be able to find the peace, joy, and happiness you were seeking in the first place.

The Way of the Samurai

At the beginning of spiritual practice, people sometimes think that they must now always put others first, making no attempt to take care of themselves. This is dangerous. The rule is: Love your neighbor *as yourself*. Self-love is the foundation for loving anyone else. If you do not love yourself, what will you have to give to another person that could possibly be of use?

This is particularly true in the realm of work. It is not only your right, but even your duty to take care of yourself. If you allow others at work to walk all over you, to destroy your peace of mind, in the name of being a good Buddhist or a good Christian or a spiritual person, you will not help them. And you will suffer a great deal. And as a consequence of your suffering and unhappiness, your family and friends and all who love you will suffer, too. You will no longer be a happy person who can offer joy and peace to those around you.

A good spiritual model here is the samurai warrior. The samurai performs his duty impersonally. He fights by following with deep awareness the flow of spiritual energy in his mind, body, and environment. If he personalizes the fight or gets angry or scared, he loses his edge. If someone succeeds in making a samurai take it personally, so that he becomes angry, by the samurai code he must withdraw from the battle in humiliation. Likewise, standing up for yourself in a work situation is not a matter of anger or personal vendetta. It is your duty to stand up for yourself. It may be paradoxical that you must stand up to the very people you include in your metta meditation, but the spiritual life is full of paradoxes. For life itself refuses to be reduced to our linear, one-dimensional thought processes.

An example comes from the Hindu devotional classic the Bhagavad Gita. As the Gita opens, Arjuna stands beside Krishna, an enlightened being and an incarnation of God, surveying the field where a great battle is about to take place. Arjuna protests that he will not fight. To fight will involve slaughtering his own kinsmen, and he will have none of it. But what does Krishna say? Krishna takes him to task for this attitude. He has to fight, he tells Arjuna, because it is his duty to do so. In the background is the fact that Arjuna belongs to the warrior caste, and it is therefore his special responsibility to fight. We do not need to take this in the sense of literal violence, of course. Mahatma Gandhi's greatest spiritual inspiration was the Gita, and he was dedicated to nonviolence. The main point is that, in whatever situation we find ourselves, we must do our duty, performing it without rancor or vengeance on the one hand, or fear and anxiety on the other. The way is to do what needs doing with nonattachment.

If you are a working person, it is your duty to do your work, and to do it in a way that does not cause injury to self or others. All working people have this responsibility, this spiritual duty. And you cannot use your spirituality to avoid standing up for yourself when that is what is called for.

The duty to take care of and defend yourself and your well-being is not a matter of becoming a steamroller that mercilessly flattens everything in its path. It is not a matter of becoming selfish, or ignoring the needs of others. But if you practice universal love and compassion, why would that not apply equally to yourself? Are you not also a part of the universe, as deserving as any other part? The Buddha taught: "You can search the tenfold universe and not find a single being more worthy of loving kindness than yourself." If you do not stand up for yourself, if you allow yourself to be abused, then your suffering will strike you at your most vulnerable point. And for people with a history of addiction, this can mean relapse.

To deal with difficult work situations and difficult people at work, you must be kind. You must also be kind to yourself. You practice metta meditation toward people at work, including the difficult ones, not only for their sake, but perhaps even more so for your own sake, so that you do not allow them to rob you of your greatest wealth—your compassion. Metta meditation for difficult people heals and helps no one so much as your own self. Yet at the same time, you must fight the fight that is before you, even if, like Arjuna, you would have none of it.

How Much Is Enough?

There is an unspoken assumption in Western culture that more is always better, that one should always be trying to seek expanding markets, to earn more and more. But this is not always conducive to peace. In contrast, consider the example of John Woolman, the Quaker tailor from Mt. Holly, New Jersey. Working at his tailoring business with peace and integrity, his work of course was of high quality and in much demand. However, when he had enough business, Woolman would simply refer people to his competitors. This allowed him time to pursue his spiritual practice and his active opposition to slavery.

Woolman knew how much was enough. We commend this koan to your practice for you to look into deeply: *How much is enough?* It is more important than meditating on the sound of one hand clapping. Do not always assume that more is better. Psychological research shows that, beyond a certain minimum, there is little relationship between wealth and happiness. Perhaps this is in part because, while wealth can bring many obvious blessings, it can be more than balanced out when we destroy our own well-being in its pursuit.

Supportive Practices

1. It has been said of Protestant reformer Martin Luther that he prayed for one hour every morning, unless of course he had a particularly busy and demanding day. In that case, he prayed for two hours.

When we are pressed and pushed by many forces, it is more important then than at any other time that we connect with the internal resources that allow us to function in the face of difficulties. Be sure that you begin your workday by connecting with your mindfulness, your peace.

If you think that you do not have time, try this: Stand facing the rising sun, and, breathing in and out, think of where you will be three hundred years from now. See the problems of the day before you in this light. Out of this insight, let laughter arise from your belly, gently at first, and then growing into great guffaws. This can be as good as hours of sitting meditation.

2. During the day, seek as many creative ways as you can to reconnect with the mindfulness that you touched in the morning. Instead of a coffee break—which will only pump you with caffeine and make your more nervous—take a "breather." Find a few minutes to breathe in and out consciously, and enjoy your breathing. Reconnect with the laughter you touched earlier, remembering the perspective of three hundred years.

You can reconnect with mindfulness at other times than formal breaks as well. When the phone rings, pause to breathe. When you complete one small task, instead of rushing on to the next, pause and breathe, enjoying two or three breaths before continuing. It requires little time to do this.

I like to leave a little time between appointments with clients to breathe and smile, to let go of the previous session and be fresh and clear for the next person. It is both a matter of self-care, and as always, at the same time, probably the best thing I could do for my clients as well.

3. In these days of *Dilbert* cubicles, it may be difficult to protect your space, but do whatever you can in this regard. If you have your own office and can close your door from time to time, do so. See if you

can teach people through this signal (and by appropriate explanation) when you are available and when you need some undisturbed space. Fill your space with green, living things if you can to evoke a sense of the natural world, and with photographs of those you love. And when you can, practice breathing in and out, looking at the plant or photo, and saying to yourself, "I know you are still with me, and I am so happy!" If you can do this deeply, the person or plant will become startlingly real to you. You will realize you have been living as if in a dream. For happiness is the power that enables each of us to contact the deepest reality.

4. See if you can use music to create your own sense of personal space and peace. Beverly loves to bring CDs from home to play quietly on her computer while she is working at her job, putting her in touch with the rest of her life. Emphasize music that is calm and healing.

5. If someone says or does something to upset you at work, take care of it and the feelings it brings up for you (see also the suggestions in the next Doorway chapter for the care of negative feelings). Do not try to deny what has happened. Sometimes when we are upset by a harsh reality, our awareness clouds over and becomes unclear and fuzzy. This is a kind of dissociated state. Try to be aware when this is happening. And when you find yourself dissociating a little from stressful events, see if you can gently begin to face them in the power of mindfulness. Then, without dismissing any painful feelings, you can return to your breathing and smiling.

When It's Time to Leave

If a work situation is causing you too much distress, robbing you of peace and well-being, or affecting your health and your relationships with those you love, it may be time to move on. It is important to handle these transition times mindfully.

Some people are tempted to make a dramatic departure, to quit on the spot when they feel mistreated in some way. Such a moment of high drama can be very satisfying in the short run, but generally it will create more problems afterward. Self-love in this instance includes slowing yourself down enough to form a plan, and having something else to go to before you leave. Otherwise, you will increase your suffering rather than decrease it.

Others are prone to stay too long. Perhaps their security needs are so great that the risk of moving on feels too frightening. Or perhaps they simply get stuck. This also is problematic. But if you are afraid or stuck, practice loving kindness and understanding toward yourself. Remember that you work in order to support a happy life. Work is not an end in itself, even if you love what you do. Your life is bigger than your job. *No job should be allowed to destroy you. Ever.*

The first part of wisdom in leaving a job is to know yourself. If you are tempted by the impulsive and dramatic sudden departure, most of the time this is not the most constructive solution. You will have to work with yourself to find ways to maintain your peace and mindfulness while you construct an alternative. If, on the other hand, you are prone to stay too long, you will also have to cultivate peace and well-being sufficient to help you get moving, make the necessary plans, begin the job search, and leave when you find a good opportunity to do so.

If your job causes you a lot of suffering, of course, it is often easier to try to do something to change it directly before you decide you need to leave. Have you worked with metta meditation for yourself and your coworkers? Have you faced your duty to stand up for yourself with some skill and grace, to try to make the situation better? These are important first steps.

Make sure to avoid romantic notions of being so spiritual that you will somehow change the atmosphere around you when this is not possible. We have pointed out that even Christ could perform no miracles in the face of extremely negative environments. And if that applied to him, it surely applies to us. Face the reality directly, mindfully. If you are the only one who is trying, the only one practicing the way of understanding and peace, and there are many others who do not care, who continually pollute the psychospiritual environment around you with toxins, with anger and power struggles and gossip and other such poisons, do not imagine that you will change such a place. Make a plan. Leave.

Further, when you are looking for a job, of course you will be concerned about what type of work it is, salary, benefits, vacation time, and so on. And these are all important. At the same time, we would urge that you also consider how happy the people who work there seem to be, and count this to be as of at least equal importance with those other things. It is helpful to sense this by having your antennae up when you are in the potentially new workplace, letting yourself feel the atmosphere there. Do people seem happy, especially when they don't know they're being observed? The atmosphere you work in will have profound effects on your well-being.

Work is a highly important aspect of our lives. It must be handled with great mindfulness. When this part of our lives is not going well, it will grab us at our most vulnerable point, possibly putting us at risk for relapse or other problems. The world needs people who can transform their work into mindfulness practice. It also needs people who do not sacrifice their own happiness to a destructive, toxic workplace. The well-being of all of us depends on this.

Doorway Nine
TRANSFORMING NEGATIVE EMOTIONS

Since everything is none other than exactly as it is,
one may well just break out in laughter.
                                    —Long Chen Pa

∽o∾

*Learn to hold and embrace difficult emotions to ensure successful
recovery. There are well-established methods for dealing with difficult feelings. If you need extra help, therapy may be a useful aid.*

∽o∾

Throughout the ages there abound miraculous stories of saints
and sages. There are stories of healing, feeding the masses,
and walking on water. There are stories of foretelling events,
remembering past lives, miraculous births, flying through the air, and
being present in more than one place at the same time. But one miracle exceeds all of these: the miracle of transforming a negative mood.

Negative emotions can be a tremendous trap, an ironclad prison.
Depression colors all of our thoughts and perceptions in the same way
that adding a teaspoon of salt to a glass of water makes all of it salty.
When depressed, we have difficulty remembering pleasant events in

the past or anticipating positive things in the future. And the present moment seems bleak, gray, and unending.

Sometimes we think negative moods are a false problem, and other kinds of problems are more real and devastating. But the exact opposite is the case. Even a person who faces life-threatening cancer has hope and some moments of peace. But the depressed person has no hope at all, and the anxious person has no peace. There is no greater darkness than the darkness of a black mood.

Some actively addicted people may be attempting to medicate themselves for a negative mood. It is difficult to learn to work with emotions; it is easy to take a drink. Working with our emotions takes time; taking a drug can be practically instantaneous. Only over time does the trap begin to reveal itself, as the addictive pattern creates more and more problems, providing ever more things to be upset about. These in turn make for an even stronger desire to escape through substance abuse, and so on in an ever-deepening downward spiral.

But even people who have become addicted for reasons other than self-medication of negative moods may lose the capacity to deal with these troubling mental states. When you quit an addiction, it can be like facing difficult feelings head on for the first time. At best, you may be out of practice at caring for negative feelings; at worst, your addiction may have created additional causes of such feelings. Part of human development is the art of emotional self-regulation, so that, unlike when we were children, it now takes a little more than a lost lollipop to make us cry. But addicted individuals may be arrested in this area of development during the time of the addiction, and are often in the position of having to learn the art of self-regulation from scratch. Since addiction is a form of avoidance, the opposite of mindfulness, then one of the things the addicted person has been avoiding is negative emotions. The bill for this neglect is now overdue.

So where do you begin? How do you start to face the challenge of negative moods and feelings? For one thing, remember again what the Buddha said: "You can search the tenfold universe and not find a single being more worthy of loving kindness than yourself." Let this idea penetrate deeply. How can you transform a negative mood, if you do not first value yourself—if you do not feel you are worthy of loving kindness? There is no one more deserving than you. *No one.*

After taking in the truth of your own worthiness, then you are
ready to transform your negative emotions. There are two basic kinds
of strategies: the cultivation of positive emotions, and the care of negative ones.

Cultivating the Positive

I vividly recall as a young man watching older adults cry in their beer
as they listened to Nat King Cole advise them to smile even if their
hearts were breaking. Already influenced by psychology and its ways
of thinking, I saw this as notoriously bad advice. To follow Cole's
advice was to commit two egregious psychological sins: denial and,
worse still, inauthenticity. The music of the decades around my birth
and prior to it were filled with such hopeful, positive messages.
Whether we were being told to accentuate the positive, or remember
our favorite things when we were sad, these were sentiments far
removed from my own. And I disdained them all.

I was wrong. While it is true that we should not deny or ignore
negative feelings, and we need to be aware of them so we can take
good care of them and transform them, we can also care for them by
cultivating positive awareness, by paying attention to the many aspects
of our current situation that are healing and wonderful, but which we
tend to take for granted. Two doors opened me to this new awareness.

The first door was not Western psychology, but Buddhist psychology. In Buddhist psychology, we have a store consciousness wherein
we keep all potential kinds of feeling and awareness in the form of
seeds. Buddhism teaches that it is very important to water selectively.
We are to encourage the growth of positive seeds, seeds of happiness,
contentment, peace, and well-being, and take care not to encourage
the growth of the negative. You do this by paying attention to the positive things, without denying the negative, but without fostering it
either. Nat King Cole pretty much had it right.

This book contains many suggestions along these lines. Coming
into the present moment, allowing yourself to be fully aware, you can
touch many healing and nurturing things. The reality of a beautiful
plant in your meditation room, the beauty and grace of the neighbor's
cat making his rounds up your sidewalk, the taste of a warm cup of

green tea on a cold, white day, the fact that your car starts easily and carries you to work safely, and so on. In fact, positive things are literally as close as your next breath. This is in many ways the best and most powerful practice. Even if those old songs and musicals seem corny to our jaded modern ears, do not write them off.

Fooling the Brain

Deep in the brain lie several important structures that influence our emotional life—the amygdala, the hypothalamus, the whole limbic system. These structures connect "downward" to incoming sensory experience, and "upward" to the cortex—the rational, thinking part of us. This pattern of connection suggests the two major ways by which we can influence our mood and our emotions. Sometimes you can "reason" with the emotions, influencing them through a more rational perspective, challenging the distortion and exaggeration in depressive thinking or worry. This can be an effective approach, and more will be said about it later under the heading "Transform Sadness." However, in the grip of a severe mood, this can feel a little like the tail trying to wag the dog.

The second approach involves the pathway from our sensory experience up to the emotional centers. In this approach, if you provide yourself with soothing, pleasing sensations, you begin to alter the state of the emotional centers themselves. For example, if you are agitated and you take a long, warm, soothing bath, it is as if the brain receives a message from the body, "I'm experiencing soothing sensations; therefore I must be feeling calm." If you are feeling unhappy, and you practice smiling, eventually you start to feel, "I'm smiling, so I must be happy." If you are feeling low in confidence, and you adopt the bodily and mental stance of a confident person, you begin to feel confident. In other words, if you start acting as though you are in the emotional state you want to cultivate, you begin to actually feel it. This is a powerful means for influencing our emotions.

From this discussion, it should be clear that, as we have said above, the addicted person is attempting to do a good thing but in an ineffective way. Addicted behavior is an attempt to provide some positive and soothing sensations. It is also a way to alter the emotional centers of the brain, through direct, chemical means. And so far as this goes, there is nothing wrong with it per se. The problem enters because the means chosen have destructive consequences beyond the temporary relief they provide. They initiate the whole destructive, addictive cycle, where one is no longer using the addictive substance for the original reason of providing relief, but comes to use it simply to avoid withdrawal. So ultimately, trying to take care of negative feelings through drugs or alcohol is like trying to put out a fire with gasoline—it's the right idea, but the wrong liquid.

Smile until you feel happy. Breathe peacefully in and out until you feel peace. Do soothing things until you are soothed. Act confidently until you feel confident. These are important practices.

Positive Psychology

Psychology has more recently begun to explore the cultivation of positive states without considering it a form of denial or repression. The positive psychology movement emphasizes that psychology should study not only how things can go wrong, but also how things go right; learning not only about depression, but also about optimism—not only about pathology, but also about resilience. Some researchers in this area are beginning to say that positive emotions heal negative ones more thoroughly and quickly than other ways. A series of experiments by Barbara Fredrikson and colleagues at the University of Michigan involved inducing negative emotional arousal in participants and measuring the effect this had on cardiac function. When participants were allowed to watch film clips that encouraged positive emotions, their hearts recovered more quickly from the negative exposure. This is in keeping with what Buddhists have been teaching for many centuries: positive emotions actually "take care of" negative ones and heal them.

Negative emotions have ripple effects. They shut down our perceptions. We see fewer options and possibilities when we are sad or anxious. But positive emotions open us up to be able to see many possibilities. In this way, positive emotions build on themselves. Things seem more possible, and so we take action more easily. We try new things and new ways of doing old things, and when some of these produce positive results, we have even more reason to feel happy. The experience of depressed people, on the other hand, is quite different.

A Vat of Thick Glue

When Larry stopped using, he found there was another problem. He was depressed. Everything in his life seemed to require immense effort. The thought of just inviting a friend to go to the movies with him seemed daunting. First of all, if he called, his friend probably would not be home. He would have to leave a message. And then, since he was going out himself, Larry probably would not be at home when his friend called back. And what if his friend did not call him right away? Worse still, what if he got some kind of obvious or mundane excuse—"Oh, I can't go. I've got to stay home and pay my bills." All of this was like walking through a vat of thick glue. It just was not worth it.

A few months later, when Larry's mood had improved, he remembered his reluctance to call his friend, which I had processed with him in therapy. Just the other day, he reported, he had called a friend to go to a movie. The friend was home, and was glad to go. Larry discovered that somehow he could just do it. It no longer required a major effort. And because he could do it, his life was now broadening out rather than narrowing. He was starting to see opportunities and possibilities where before there was only drudgery and despair.

A simple thing like going to the movies with a friend gets you moving, and helps you open to life's positive possibilities. Nothing much positive can happen while you sit around and worry or feel sad.

Taking Care of the Negative

None of what has been said above should be construed as denial or repression. It is simply the case that sometimes we can take care of negative emotions simply by tuning in more deeply to the positive elements of our experience. You are not trying to avoid the negative or deny that such feelings exist. It is like taking care of your tomato plants. There are simply two kinds of things that you need to do. One is to attend to the weeds, to take them out so that your plants are not strangled in competition for resources. The other is to care directly for the plants themselves, providing the sunshine, water, and soil nutrients needed for growth. If you can do this directly with your tomato plants (positive feelings), they will be stronger and better able to handle the competition with the weeds (negative feelings).

However, sometimes we must weed our garden also. We must pull the weeds out so our tomatoes can grow. Even so, we can use the weeds for compost. We do not just try to get rid of them. Negative emotions are us, and we are our negative emotions. If we try to just get rid of them, we are trying to get rid of ourselves. This is indeed the approach of denial and repression, and it simply does not work in the long run. We have to find ways to work with these feelings directly, and transform them rather than discard them.

Transform Sadness

The first step in dealing with a negative emotion is the cultivation of calmness—in Buddhist teaching, *samatha*. If you are feeling sad, this is not so bad. You can work with sadness. But when there is an element of agitation along with the sadness, it becomes difficult to find your way. Sadness in its pure form can be transformed. But if you are also telling yourself that it is terrible to have this feeling, and it must stop, *Now!*—then you do not have sufficient calm and perspective.

So the first step is to find a way to calm down. You can do this by breathing in and out, giving your attention to the breathing and to the sadness you are feeling, holding the sadness as you would a crying infant, smiling to it. You would not handle a crying baby by thrusting it away or being angry with it in turn, scolding it to "grow up." If you did, the baby would become even more agitated. Instead you help a crying baby by rocking it, cooing to it or singing, letting it feel the calm rhythm of your beating heart and the soothing wavelike motion of your breathing. If you have been using conscious breathing in your meditation, so that it already triggers feelings of calm and peace, it will be available to you when you need it to calm and take care of negative feelings.

Be aware of all that you are feeling and thinking, and how these emotions play themselves out in your body as well—that tightness in the neck and shoulders, a tension in the belly. Whatever you notice, just breathe in and out with these feelings and sensations.

There is a balancing act here. It is much like the mother with the crying infant. If the mother identifies too much with the baby's pain, she will become distraught herself. Then contact with the mother will not be soothing to the baby, but will amplify the baby's distress. An amplifying feedback loop gets started, such that the upset baby causes the mother to feel upset, and when the baby feels the mother's distress, he becomes even more distressed, which distresses the mother even more, and so on. But neither will it do for the mother to say to herself, "There's that baby, crying again. I'll just leave him alone to work it out on his own." Babies cannot do this alone. They lack the cognitive development required for emotional regulation. They need the mother's help.

Likewise, your negative feelings need to be held by your mindfulness. In learning to calm your own feelings of sadness or distress, you need to strike a balance, being neither too detached (which is denial or repression) nor too involved. It is as though you hold the emotions with great tenderness, but without going inside them, not identifying with them to such a degree that you lose yourself in them.

If you pay attention to what happens to your breathing when you are upset, you will notice that such emotions affect your breathing dramatically. Breathing comes in short gasps and gets caught. It becomes shallow, rapid, irregular. As you begin to pay attention to your breathing, it naturally begins to smooth out and deepen, without any particular effort from you. Smooth, slow breathing such as occurs when we breathe consciously is associated with feelings of calm and ease. Psychology calls this an incompatible response. Just as it is difficult to both smile and be sad at the same time, so it is also difficult to continue to be agitated when your breath is smooth, regular, and deep. In a sense, conscious breathing is itself the maternal presence that calms your agitation. Even a few minutes of this practice can help a lot—not perhaps making your sadness disappear all at once, but certainly calming the agitation that prevents insight and healing.

Once you have established some calmness, you can begin to look into the nature of the sadness you are feeling. When the waves of your thoughts and emotions have become more tranquil, you can then look down into the water and see what lies below the surface. This is not so much a matter of trying to dissect and analyze your situation logically as it is of allowing the insight to emerge of its own accord, without forcing it. It is a little like the paradox found in the teaching of the Course in Miracles, which states that absolute patience brings instant results. When you are not trying to force it, insight comes. This attitude is expressed wonderfully in the Zen teaching:

Sitting quietly, doing nothing,
Spring comes, and the grass grows by itself.
Insight likewise comes of itself,
ripening and falling from the tree of mindfulness.

You might notice that the feeling of sadness you carry is related to your upbringing. A parent who is perpetually worried about money can infect a child with this same fear and uneasiness, becoming a kind of self-fulfilling prophecy that creates the very thing that is feared. Or it may be that you realize that the origins of your sadness lie in some crucial empathic failure on the part of your parents, something you desperately needed from them but did not get. If you look deeply into your sadness, you do not have to be stuck with just blaming your parents, however. Blaming your parents is just substituting one kind of disease for another—in this case, substituting anger and blame for sadness. But continue to look more deeply until you can also see that your parents inherited their limitations from their parents and other life experiences.

The Bible says that the sins of the fathers shall be passed on to the sons unto the third and fourth generation. As a statement of justice, this is horribly unfair. But as a psychological truth, it is undeniable. We pass on our own problems and blind spots, our pain and worry, to our children. In this way, taking care of our negative feelings is a gift not only to ourselves, but to future generations.

You may also notice certain things about the quality of your thinking when you are depressed. Depressive thinking exaggerates. Depressive thinking tends, for one thing, to be black and white, seeing only the extremes, missing all the shades of gray. Depression loves words like *always* and *never*: "I *never* get what I want. I *always* mess things up. Things *never* turn out the way I hope."

Depressive thinking minimizes our good points, and exaggerates our shortcomings. A single mistake becomes an unending pattern of failure and defeat, while we hardly think twice about positive aspects of who we are and what we have accomplished. We are invariably to blame for things that turn out badly, but anything that succeeds is a matter of sheer luck.

See if you can identify these distorted elements in your sad thinking, and try to gently substitute a more realistic thought. "I never do anything right!" becomes "It's true I made a mistake, but everyone does from time to time. I do some good things, too." And "I'm a no-good loser" becomes "You win some, you lose some. That's life."

However, remember the principle of not forcing. Be gentle with these insights. And, of course, do not let them be another vehicle for self-reproach: "What a jerk I am! I *always* exaggerate!"

As you look deeply into sad feelings, you may also notice something else. You may notice that there can be a kind of guilty pleasure in feeling sad, a reveling in the very bitterness that you feel. You may see that you are resisting cultivating positive feelings because then you would have to give up this very enjoyable sadness. Besides, viewing things more positively and less distortedly would mean also losing your right to be upset, and losing your freedom to act irresponsibly for a time. "How can you expect *me* to be concerned about doing the dishes, when I am in such a crisis?"

The most important practice is to look into these things lovingly, with absolute acceptance for the way you are at this time. Buddhists talk about the idea of no self. This does not mean you do not exist, but that you are a composite. You are made of materials that are not you—water, minerals, and proteins, as well as experiences and memories. When you see this condition deeply, you know you are not to blame. Anyone with your genes and your life experiences would be feeling the same emotional storm you are in right now. *But while you are not to blame, you are responsible.* That is, you can choose how you *respond* to the situation you are in. You can make the choice to do something to take care of negative feelings and transform them.

Of course, you cannot just flip a switch and turn your sadness off. That is what the addicted person tries to do with drugs. But while there is no switch, you do have a lot of influence. By breathing, calming, and looking deeply, you create a context in which healing can take place. The healing, however, comes of itself, in the same way that you digest food or grow hair or fingernails without thinking.

Deal with Worry and Anxiety

Our modern world is full of schedules and structures. We set deadlines and appointment times in order to ensure that the work gets done in a reasonable amount of time, and that we meet each other at the right place and time. But every deadline becomes a source of worry. Will I get it done by then? Am I making reasonable progress, or falling behind? And every appointment time contributes to our anxiety. Did I note the time and place correctly? Will I forget? What if the other person doesn't remember?

The speed at which we move is in itself anxiety producing. We do not move at the pace of our innate organic rhythms, but at car speed and jet speed. We are always moving on to the next thing, trying to arrive rather than travel. We are so goal directed and purposive that we never stop to live—which in itself creates a constant background of worry and fear. "Paradoxical as it may seem," commented Alan Watts in *The Way of Zen* (1957), "the purposeful life has no content, no point. It hurries on and on, and misses everything. Not hurrying, the purposeless life misses nothing—for it is only when there is no goal and no rush that the human senses are fully open to receive the world."

Anxiety and worry can also be a signal that we are living in a way that is inauthentic—which is perhaps to say the same thing somewhat differently. When we are not being genuine—when too much of our energy goes into trying to figure out who we need to be for others to like us or just to get along in the world, without paying sufficient attention to who we really are and what we really want—we feel uneasy. There is a sense that somehow this is all wrong and out of kilter, out of balance and out of Tao.

In addition, some people have more sensitive nervous systems than others. While some are relatively calm by temperament, others are more reactive. The events of daily life reverberate in endless echoes through the mind, body, and emotions of such people. This obviously creates more worry, particularly in the modern world where a forced, mechanical beat replaces the organic, lunar, and solar rhythms of the ancients. But such sensitivity can also be a blessing. People with oversensitive nervous systems cannot fool themselves as long, cannot continue living inauthentically without paying a heavy price. Such people are forced to listen, to pay attention to what is happening with them. And in this sense, many of the people seen in therapy have an advantage over those who are walking around outside without knowing or recognizing their own suffering.

What if we told you that there is a Buddhist practice that can eliminate fear, worry, and anxiety from your daily life? Would we have your attention?

There is such a practice.

PRACTICE

The Five Remembrances

Spend some time each morning breathing in and out, and looking deeply into each of the following truths. You might like to coordinate the words in parentheses with your breath, saying the first phrase with your inbreath, and the second one with your outbreath.

1. I am of a nature to grow old. I cannot escape old age. (growing old, no escape)
2. I am of a nature to suffer ill health. I cannot escape ill health. (ill health, no escape)
3. I am of a nature to die. I cannot escape death. (death, no escape)
4. Everything and everyone I love is of a nature to change. I cannot hold on to any of them. (everything changes, losing everything)
5. My deeds (karma) are my only true possessions. (deeds, true possessions)

Spend enough time on each point to contact the reality. Avoid just saying the words without insight. Do not use this practice if you are sad; just as you do not get a flu shot when you have the flu.

Can you see how this practice leads to no fear? If you know the full reality that you will die—if you see it clearly, and not as some vague notion of something that occurs to other people but not to ourselves—this normally unpalatable fact can liberate you from worry and fear. In the face of this truth, what is there, ultimately, that is worth worrying about? It only makes sense to worry when we believe that we live this life forever. When we contact the reality of death, we no longer need to dwell in anxiety.

Sometimes people feel that this practice is too negative. They may even have a superstitious attitude toward it, as though thinking about such negative things would somehow bring them on. But as we have argued, more harm comes from not facing the reality of our lives than comes from facing it. Even if you believe in an afterlife or reincarnation, it is nonetheless true that *this* life, as we know it, is limited and does come to an end. No harm will befall you from facing the truth. And what seems like a negative practice becomes a source of joy and liberation, and fear decreases.

Paradoxically, pretending we will never die leads to greater anxiety, because we are trying to deny the obvious reality. Seeing this reality head on frees us, relativizes our daily struggle, allowing us to enjoy the many wonders present here and now in this moment of living awareness.

No escaping old age. Technically, of course, this is not completely true. You may not live to old age. But as the old joke has it, even though we may not like aging, we like the alternative even less. This involves looking old age straight in the face as something that will happen and in fact is happening to us already, right now. It is nothing abstract. It is real and concrete. Nor is it something that only happens to other people. One fruit of this practice is that you see older people a little differently.

No escaping ill health. It is true of course that some people may not experience a prolonged period of great incapacitation. But all of us suffer ill health to some extent. Which one of us has never caught a cold, or suffered a headache or a toothache? The idea of perfect health is just that—an idea. It is not real. At every moment, every one of us falls short of this artificial concept. We are always repairing some minor difficulty, some cut or bruise or hangnail. Knowing that we cannot escape ill health, we learn to enjoy the many elements of health that are present now.

No escaping death. This is the heart of it. Old age and illness are only preludes to this one. Death is not just a concept, and it is not just something that happens to other people. Think of all the billions of human beings who lived before us, each of them valuing his or her existence as much as we do ours, each of them in the end succumbing to death. Where are they now? Where will you be in a few hundred years? Look at this straight on. These very bones that you can touch and feel through your own skin will as surely become dust as those of ancient humans and prehumans and nonhumans.

If you deny this fact, you get caught in the wheel of suffering, endlessly pursuing more wealth, more security, more love and recognition. But where does it all end? Nowhere! You become like people drinking salt water to quench your thirst—each sip creates more of the very thing that is the problem.

We knew a man who was ninety years old and was very wealthy. He complained to me one day when he had to travel to a city five hundred miles away that the airfares were too high. And so, at ninety years of age, he and his wife drove the whole way instead.

You know the end of the story already, because in one form or another, it is the end of all stories: one day he suddenly had a stroke, and within a day or two, he died. Now where are his millions? Would it not have been better if he had enjoyed his wealth more fully, instead of pretending that he was in an unending life game of trying to amass more and more?

Seeing clearly into the inevitability of death is enhanced when it is not just an isolated meditation exercise, but a daily reminder of reality. When a business deal falls through, when someone whose respect or admiration you hope for insults you instead, when someone aggravates you with her aggressive driving, when someone cancels an appointment with you at the last minute, or whatever happens that tends to frustrate or aggravate you, making you sad or despairing or angry—that moment is a perfect time to remind yourself of your final destination.

The result of acknowledging death is fullness of life. When you see that this will happen to you, that it is inevitable and that only the time is uncertain, what is there to fear?

No Self, No Problem

Ralph Waldo Emerson wrote: "A foolish consistency is the hobgoblin of little minds." When we are experiencing a negative emotion, one of the ways in which we create difficulties is by then trying to be consistent with ourselves. If I am angry at you, but you do something that makes me want to laugh, you may witness an extraordinarily contorted facial expression. Because there is a part of me that feels: "I'm angry, I shouldn't laugh."

From a Buddhist perspective, this is the problem of clinging to the idea of self. One of the ways we continue to assert the illusion of a self is through just such consistency. If we allowed our mood to change and flow freely, in accord with its own nature, how could we feel we were the same person from day to day, or even from moment to moment? Being consistent, even with negative and destructive behaviors, consoles us that we are the same person as ever. If we just changed freely from moment to moment, we might be confronted with the terrifying fact of change and impermanence. We might be confronted with a sense of ourselves that feels much less solid than we would like.

The Buddhist way is to embrace impermanence and no self. For if you try to tune into just where your "self" is, all you will find ultimately is an ever-changing flow of experience. The idea of a self is just one part of the flow.

Holding on to a solid sense of self creates great difficulties. If we are sad, we must stay sad. If we are worried, we must stay worried. But if you tune in to the flow of experience, and cease straining against it, you can laugh when someone does something funny—even if you have been feeling angry. You don't have to hold on so tightly: no self, no problem.

PRACTICE

The Four Noble Truths

Buddhist teachings are not really a philosophy or a theology. They are a way of life, a practice. This applies to the core of the Buddha's teaching as well. The Four Noble Truths—suffering, the cause of suffering, the way out of suffering, and the path of well-being—are a practice.

The first truth is that suffering is. When you suffer, when you are unhappy, the most important step is the first one—to recognize that you are suffering. You can do nothing about your suffering if you do not allow yourself to recognize it. So when you are suffering, acknowledge it. That is the first step. Breathe in and out, and smile to your suffering, for by smiling you assert your capacity to be mindful.

The second truth is that suffering has a cause. When you look deeply into reality, calming yourself, you can see what is really causing your suffering. Often this is not what you think. It is not the circumstances or people you want to blame. It is yourself. The question is not what others have done to you to get you into this mess. The question is, What are you doing that creates your suffering? How are you living?

The third truth is that there is a way out. This is easy once you have identified the factors that are causing your suffering. Once you know the true cause, it is easy to see what you need to do.

The fourth truth—The Eightfold Path of Right View, Right Thinking, Right Speech, and so on—is an explication of the path of well-being. If there is a correct way to think, speak, act, work, and so on, then there are ways that are incorrect, which cause suffering rather than alleviate it.

Whenever you suffer, calm yourself, and use the Four Noble Truths as your guide. Recognize your suffering. Inquire into its nature, its causes. Ask yourself what you are doing that creates the suffering, and what you need to do to find well-being. When you have some insight, talk to a trusted friend about it, and see if she can add to it.

None Other Than the Way It Is

At this point we can return to the quotation from Long Chen Pa in the epigraph of this Doorway: Everything is just so. Why not laugh? How absurd it is to go on striving and fighting! It is even more absurd to fight our tendency to fight, instead of seeing this also as a fact of nature, a storm, a cypress tree, or a mountain.

There are two common objections that may be raised to this profound teaching of Long Chen Pa. First of all, if we just take things as they are, won't we be in danger of becoming too passive, not doing what we can to improve our lot and the lot of others? Is such indifference really the way? And second, isn't such laughter inevitably bitter and cynical? Will it not ring hollow and empty?

We imagine these objections to be valid because of the persistent habit of our divided minds. We cannot imagine the profound acceptance behind such a teaching. For us, acceptance inevitably is held in tension with nonacceptance, peace in tension with struggle, joy with sadness. But what Buddhist teaching points to is an acceptance, a peace, a joy that is inclusive rather than exclusive. It is like the wide, blue, New Mexican sky. It contains easily and effortlessly all the birds and planes and clouds that pass through it. Likewise, the reason that mindfulness does not lead to too passive an attitude toward life is that our tendency to take action is included in it rather than ruled out. Taking action is simply another aspect of things being just as they are.

Experience also teaches that such laughter is not cynical or hollow. Cynicism is the result of resisting, of not really accepting things fully just as they are. But all of us have experiences quite different from this. All of us have stood before a gold-streaked sunset or ocean panorama with simple awe, taking it in just as it is, smiling in secret joy, having no need to tell anyone else about it or use it in any way, just being there, just enjoying it for its own sake.

One way to express this is to draw a distinction between happiness and joy, between what might be called quietude and peace, between trading and love. Happiness, at least as the word is used here, is a function of what *happens* to us. Happiness is dependent on circumstances. When you get the new job, pass the test, find the person you want to love and be with forever, you feel happiness. But joy is something else. Joy is that feeling that wells up inside you for no reason at all. If quietude is dependent on having serene external circumstances, then true peace is something that arises in us independently of that. Similarly, when we are simply attuned to other people with mindfulness and understanding, love and compassion arise. We then engage in loving action—not as an investment on which we hope someday to receive a return, but simply because this is the thing to do, because we have touched the reality of the other person.

Joy, peace, and love are realities that are always there and that need no particular circumstance or any special effort to become manifest. When our vision is clear, we can touch them at any time. When we touch them, we touch the reality of the universe all around us more deeply. And when we touch the universe deeply, we touch joy, peace, and love. They simply are.

Your smile shows that you know just what this means.

Things to Do When Negative Emotions Strike

1. Return to your breathing. Embrace and accept the feeling just as it is, holding it and calming it.

2. Look deeply into these feelings. As you begin to feel a little more calm, see what insight comes up for you about being in this circumstance—how it came to be, what the way out is. Allow these insights to arise without forcing.

3. See if you can find an element of distortion or exaggeration in your thoughts. Be present with these in a gentle, loving way, without fighting with them. See if more positive and constructive ways of thinking emerge.

4. See the troubling event or circumstance in light of the Five Remembrances. See if laughter wells up.

5. Practice walking meditation. There is something soothing about the rhythmic motion of walking, the fresh air, the contact with the outside world. If you are also cultivating awareness of the present moment and appreciation of the walking and the many wonders around you, doing your best not to just rehearse your worries, half an hour or an hour of this practice can be *incredibly* helpful.

6. If you engage in distraction, engage in it mindfully (without worrying about the paradox). If you watch a movie, try to be as present to it as you can. Take it in deeply. Perhaps you also want to take some care to pick one that is not too depressing or anger provoking. If you succumb to your love of chocolate, really succumb. Try not to wolf it down in the car, but instead, sit someplace where you can really enjoy the chocolate, chewing it slowly and mindfully. Enjoy it more deeply than you normally would, rather than less.

7. Call a friend who has some stability in mindfulness practice, and ask to sit beside him or her for a while.

8. Call your therapist if you have one. If you do not, and if you have a tendency to be overwhelmed by negative emotions more than you would like, find one. It's great if you can find one who is interested in mindfulness. But if not, don't worry. All therapy worthy of the name seeks to raise awareness in one way or another, and is in this sense a mindfulness practice.

9. If your emotions are triggering a desire to drink or use, remember that the worst part of this is usually over fairly quickly. Engage in some activity that will occupy your active attention for a while. By

then you may find that the urge is quite manageable. Or try being with the urge and breathing mindfully, exploring it like any other thought crossing your mind—if this is comfortable for you.

10. Remember that the same thing applies to moods: they also do not last. Allow yourself to experience a mood without fear that you will be caught there forever, since mood is as impermanent as everything else.

11. Practice active imagination. See if the present mood can be drawn, painted, danced, or written about. Perhaps the mood wants to personify itself in some inner character of your psyche, whom you can draw or engage in a written dialogue. Notice how the mood shifts.

12. Practice no self. "I am just experiencing this particular mood or emotion. It does not have to be clung to, or feared. It can settle itself."

13. Look deeply into this truth: *No one in the entire universe is more deserving of loving kindness than I am.*

Doorway Ten

LIVING MOMENT BY MOMENT

This minute that comes to me over the past decillions,
There is no better than it and now.
　　　　—Walt Whitman, "Song of Myself" (1855)

Wheresoever you turn, there is the face of God.
　　　　—Qur'an

∽◦∾

*Practice, practice, practice. An intellectual understanding of how to
change your life is just the beginning. Direct experience brings the
peace, health, and wholeness you seek.*

∽◦∾

The Good Portion

In the preceding Doorways, we have provided you with many tools
for cultivating mindfulness in daily life. If you have begun to put
these into practice, you already know that each step in the direction of mindfulness is a step toward fullness of life, peace, joy, and
understanding. As your capacity to live this way deepens, you become
a happier person. Relapse is increasingly unimaginable. When every
moment of your life is a walk in the Buddhaland, in the Kingdom of
Heaven, there is simply no need to run to the false security of drugs.

215

At the same time, having so many tools can also seem a little over-whelming—as though you had a lot of things to do and remember. It isn't so. Whenever you feel this way, it is good to remind yourself that there is really only one thing to remember, and it is the simplest thing of all: to be mindful, to be aware. Everything we have discussed is just a means to this one end. When you keep the end in mind, you will know what to do and what not to do.

In the gospel of Luke, there is a famous story about Jesus visiting two sisters. Martha was busy doing all the little things involved with running a household and receiving guests, while Mary sat and listened to Jesus. Martha got pretty sick of this after a while. She complained to Jesus about her lazy sister, who left her to do all the work.

Much has been said and written about these two sisters in Christian tradition—a lot of it arguing that Martha wasn't really so bad, and that we need people engaged in active service. That is true also. But this is what Jesus said to Martha, the busy one, about Mary:

> Martha, Martha, you are anxious and trouble about many things; *one thing is needful*. Mary has chosen the good portion, which shall not be taken away from her. (Luke 10:41–42, italics ours)

This affirmation of the contemplative approach to life is still so revolutionary that commentators rush to soften its impact, as if to protect us from the obvious absurdity of spending our lives vacantly mooning around—as though most of us were in danger on that account. Most people are in far greater danger of excessive busyness than of becoming too inactive or passive. Yet even if you have many things to do, you can learn to choose the good portion. You can learn to maintain a focus on what is really needed. And what is needed is mindfulness—this open, calm, nourishing attention, not choosing between this and that, accepting things just as you find them, letting people and situations settle themselves.

The Surfer

A great image for living mindfully is the life of a surfer. He rises early in the morning, eager to face the surf. He takes great care with his board, waxing it, handling it with love and attention. All of this may look like some bizarre ritual, but he accepts it all as a part of his endeavor. Once on the water, he shows great patience, waiting for the wave that will give him the ride he wants. He is not afraid of the waves, but faces them with confidence, trusting his capacity to ride each one. What he does has absolutely no point or utilitarian value. That is precisely what makes it so beautiful.

If you told him that what he was doing was something admirable, if you said you admired his discipline, he would look at you strangely. Riding the waves is a joy to him. So if by discipline, you mean that he is suppressing himself or restraining himself in some way from what he really wants to do, this is not the case. He is doing exactly what he wants. It is only from the outside that you could imagine there is discipline in what he is doing. It is only if you do not know the joy of riding the waves that you could think he is leading some kind of ascetic life. "The Tao [the way of life]," wrote Zen master Ma-tsu, "has nothing to do with discipline." But lest you confuse this with being lax, he adds: "If you say there is no discipline, this is to be the same as ordinary people." The way of the surfer resolves the paradox. While some might say he is a surf bum, others may admire his discipline and effort. But the surfer himself is just following the joy of blending harmoniously with the energy of the waves.

The most important thing about learning to live mindfully and cherish each moment of life is to approach mindfulness practice as a joy.

Rising Early

It might be possible to learn to live mindfully without practicing meditation, but we would not want to bet on it. Similarly, it might be possible to live a mindful, spiritual life without rising early, but the odds are against it. Perhaps you do not need to rise at 3:00 A.M. as some Buddhist monks do. But it is essential to get up early enough to allow yourself a sense of time in the morning. If you hit the ground running from the time the alarm goes off, it is very difficult from there to recover your mindfulness. Even getting up just half an hour earlier may be enough time to allow you to have a sense of spaciousness in your morning, to be able to do things without rushing, to allow at least a little while to practice meditation. When you know what a joy this is, you will not confuse it with harsh discipline. Starting the day this way makes everything go better. For if you do not touch your mindfulness at the beginning of the day, how will mindfulness be possible?

Allow time in the morning to begin your day with a sense of peace and mindfulness. Even before you get out of bed, breathe in and out a few times. For the intention is to live each moment deeply, calmly, peacefully. Allow time to be present to your breakfast, to your coffee or tea. Allow time to get to work, so that you do not destroy your mindfulness by making your drive to work a battle. Allow some time to sit and breathe mindfully, and perhaps do a page or two of inspirational reading to help set the tone for the day.

A Buddhist teaching says you should practice as though your hair were on fire. This means that once you see the truth of your situation, how you are suffering when you live in forgetfulness, you will naturally want to do something about it. A person whose hair is on fire does not need a lot of urging to find water.

Just Riding the Waves

If you touch mindfulness in the morning, it will be much easier to keep it going during the day. The events of the day are just waves. Some waves are powerful and difficult. Some are gentle and easy. While you are learning to surf, you fall off many times. But if you are enjoying yourself, you will not let this stop you. You can laugh and get right back up, touching mindfulness, regaining your balance. The next time you ride a wave like that, you will do better.

Daily life throws many difficult waves at us. Perhaps you have done your best to leave enough time for the drive to work. You drive onto the busy freeway smiling, peaceful, with a sense of freedom, because you know you do not need to fight. You can breathe in and out and smile when the traffic stops. But some days you encounter unanticipated road work. Or you encounter a major accident, which slows you down and makes you late for work. Your blood pressure starts to rise. You start to upset yourself, thinking, "This is terrible! This can't be! I'll be late, and I *can't* be late!" But if you come back to yourself enough so that you can smile and breathe and stop fighting even a little bit, you are cultivating mindfulness. And your capacity to be mindful increases. As you become mindful, you remember that the road work is difficult but necessary for all of us. You have compassion for the workers who must do this difficult work, made dangerous by the presence of so many cars with so many impatient drivers. You remember that the accident may be much more than an annoyance to the people involved in it, perhaps injuring them or killing them, maybe changing their lives forever. Suddenly you can be glad that all you are facing is the prospect of being late for work. Each time you do your best to work mindfully with your feelings of frustration or pressure, you increase your capacity to meet other difficult moments with equanimity.

Joyful Waves

But riding difficult waves is only part of the truth. While it is vital to be in touch with these difficult aspects, it is just as important to be in touch with the wonderful waves that come along and give you a wonderful ride toward the shore. In mindfulness practice, this is nothing rare. But as you slow down and open up to your life, you know more and more that wonderful things are all around you, all the time. And being in contact with these wonderful things gives you the strength to be mindful in the difficult things.

PRACTICE

Imagine Nothing

Sit somewhere quiet, preferably where you have a nice view. Breathe in and out and close your eyes. After a few moments, when you have centered and calmed yourself, imagine *nothing*. Try intensively to imagine nothing. Go ahead. Do this for a few minutes before you go on to the next paragraph.

How did you do? Chances are, in trying to think about nothing, you pictured something like a blackness, a void, empty space. However, blackness and space are something in themselves. So try again. Think about *nothing*. Do this for a few minutes again before reading on.

Now as you open your eyes, see how wonderful it is that there is *something*. You take it for granted, but something is there all the time. Isn't it wonderful?

Before you react, before you divide the world into things that are pleasant or unpleasant, things you like or dislike, there is just the world. There is just *something*. It is neither good nor bad, but all of it is wonderful when you realize that there is no necessity for there to be something. It just is. It's a gift. It's grace.

Seeing things this way changes your relationship to everything, including difficult people. If you imagine them not existing, as though they had never been born, there is a sense of loss. And it is not just the positive aspects of this person that would be a loss. If you take this seriously, even their more difficult aspects would be a loss. Difficult people complicate our lives in interesting ways, and if they are unpleasant ways, they are yet wonderful ways.

To catch even a glimpse of this truth is to touch Buddhahood.

Every Wave Is a Wonderful Wave

Einstein said there are two ways of looking at the world—seeing nothing as miraculous, or seeing everything as miraculous. To see everything as miraculous frees you to enjoy every moment. You no longer have to pick and choose between moments you like and those you dislike. When you see more deeply, every wave is wonderful, whether it is good for surfing or not. Everything that happens is wonderful when no longer seen exclusively through the narrow lens of what meets or thwarts your purposes.

The more you cultivate this kind of awareness, the easier it becomes to be deeply in each moment. To be grateful that there is something, when there could be nothing, is to touch the miracle of creation. Then every day is the first day, fresh and clear and clean. No day is wasted.

Consider the Lilies

In a famous Buddhist story, the Buddha held a flower silently before a large gathering of his monks. Finally one of them, Mahakashyapa, smiled at the Buddha. The Buddha said he had transmitted an insight to Mahakashyapa. People have speculated endlessly about what sort of mystical truth was exchanged between them. But it is simpler than that. (It always is, and enlightenment itself hides from us only because it is the simplest thing of all.) Mahakashyapa got it because *he was the one who saw the flower*.

"Do not be anxious. . . . Consider the lilies, how they grow; they neither toil nor spin; yet I tell you, even Solomon in all his glory was not arrayed like one of these" (Luke 6:25, 28). In a letter to a friend, Emily Dickinson said that considering the lilies was the only commandment she never broke. From a mindfulness perspective, it is an excellent choice.

Obstacles

Mindfulness is simple. It is the simplest thing in the world. It is not always easy, but if you bring intelligence and gentle persistence to this path, you will find you can do it, too.

In the movie *The Edge*, Anthony Hopkins played the part of a wealthy man who got lost in the Alaskan wilderness and had to face a hungry, man-killing bear. Knowing that other men had survived confrontations with bears, Hopkins's character used the mantra over and over, "What one man can do, another man can do." In the end, he killed the bear.

In Buddhism, it is stressed that the Buddha was a human being. He was a real person, like you and me, and not a god. That is why it took centuries in the Buddhist world before any statues of the Buddha appeared. The Buddhist's humanity brings out an important and encouraging truth. What one man or woman can do, another can do. You also can reach enlightenment. The life of the Buddha shows us what is possible.

Slips

For recovering people, of course, slips are the biggest obstacle of all. Using alcohol or other drugs is the opposite of mindfulness. Slips are a strong form of lapsing into forgetfulness or nonmindfulness.

Of course, slips are important and dangerous. At the same time, we feed these monsters if we think about them in too black-and-white a manner. If we divide life up into the two rigid categories of abstinent versus nonabstinent, we will not be able to be mindful of our slips in a healing way. Mindfulness means experiencing life beyond the rigid categories of our thought—pleasant/unpleasant, good/bad, abstinent/using. While some people manage to stop an addictive behavior in one fell swoop, this is rare. Most of us, in learning to change a habit, go through cycles—making mistakes, learning from them, making more mistakes, learning from them—until we become stable and solid in the new way of being.

When you let go of rigid categories, you can reflect mindfully on a slip. You can look deeply into it, learn from it, and find what you need to avoid it next time. Ask yourself, what led up to the slip? What else could I have done to prevent it? What other choices could I have made? How was I viewing the situation then, and how else could I have looked at it? If you see a slip in black-and-white terms, it is another failure experience—another indication that your situation is hopeless. But if you see it mindfully, a slip is an opportunity to learn.

Not Being Busy

Life can indeed seem overwhelming. We live with such pressure, with so many things to do. Yet if you calm down, breathe, and meditate on this problem, you will see that it need not be an obstacle. When you look deeply into your busy life, there are two kinds of truth that emerge. The solution in any particular case will involve some combination of these two answers.

The first truth is, *Simplify your life*. There are many stories of busy people who have been forced to reduce the number of things they do. Some busy chief executives who have suffered heart attacks, for example, have had to cut their workload in half. As important as these people are in their companies, they manage to do it. Yet if you had asked them before the heart attack if it would have been possible for them to do so, they would have denied it. What a shame they could not have reached this insight *before* the heart attack!

If you are mindful, you know that being busy is a choice. Look deeply into the reasons why you choose to have so much to do. Your reasons could be many. In our society, for example, it is a status symbol to be busy. Some people actually create crisis after crisis in part because it feeds a sense of self-importance, whereas if they were more mindful, if they paid attention to small matters before they became large problems, many of these crises could have been anticipated and avoided. Our cell phones announce our importance to the world, yet somehow people survived before they were invented. Some of our gadgets keep us on a constant leash, so we are never free. Some people genuinely need these things, and in other cases they may be a worthwhile convenience. But it is good to question the automatic assumption that such things always increase our quality of life. Consider. Are there ways you can become a little less available? Are there tasks you can delegate? Are there things you could really let go of? Would life on earth end if you did a little less?

Please, for the sake of your own well-being, and for the sake of others as well, be slow to conclude there is no way to reduce your workload and other forms of busyness. You may be a happier person, and contribute much more to the happiness of others, if you are less harried. Still, you may need to realize the second truth here as well.

That second truth is, *Learn the art of wu wei (nondoing)*. Nondoing is not the same as doing nothing. It means finding the peace and silence in the midst of activity and noise. Often it is not what you are doing per se that wears you out, but your inner attitude. As much as you may be doing on the outside, you are often doing much more on the inside. While you are driving, you are rehearsing a hundred things you need to remember to do and accomplish. You get exhausted not because of driving, but because of your internal busyness. No wonder you are exhausted at the end of the day. Whatever you have done and accomplished, mentally you have done countless other things.

Many saints and sages, contrary to popular opinion, have been very busy, active people. It is their spirituality that has enabled them to be so active and accomplish so much without becoming fragmented. In mindfulness practice, learn to drive when you are driving. Learn to walk when you are walking. Learn to type when you are typing. If you can be present to doing one thing at a time, you will find life a lot less tiring.

Keep Mindfulness Practice Fun

Once the Dalai Lama was to give an important, deep, esoteric teaching in New York. Before he spoke, monks chanted on the stage for hours to prepare the atmosphere spiritually. A special throne was prepared for him to sit on. When the Dalai Lama finally came out to speak, he approached his special seat. As he sat on it, the cushions gave him a slight bounce. He laughed a little, and bounced again, a childlike grin on his face. This may have been a more important teaching than the talk.

There is a tendency for us to get *serious* when it comes to spiritual practice. This is an overreaction. Of course, practice is important, and we want to avoid being frivolous about it. But it is also important to approach spiritual practice in a spirit of fun, of joy and ease.

Don't let becoming a spiritual person deprive you of a sense of humor. Humor is a spiritual gift. Find a way to practice that gives you a sense of lightness and fun.

If you are pouring yourself a cup of coffee, can you find the fun in it? If you do it in forgetfulness, there is no fun in it at all. You probably will not even taste the coffee when you drink it, let alone be present to the pouring as a valid moment in your life. Children know, however, that such things can be fun. Have you ever seen children at a make-believe tea party? They don't even need the tea to enjoy themselves.

Practice in a way that you find the fun.

Staying with It

Sometimes you may begin the day with meditation and other practices to try to live more mindfully, but quickly get sucked into the maelstrom of forgetfulness. You struggle to return to mindfulness, but cannot seem to find the way. When you look deeply into this situation, there are several factors you may want to consider.

For one thing, perhaps you have not put sufficient energy in the beginning of the day into your intention to live mindfully. As you practice your morning sitting meditation, review in your mind why you want to live more mindfully, and what it is like to live in forgetfulness. Clearly envision the difference between the mindful life and the nonmindful life. Put some energy into an intention to do your best to live with clear awareness.

For another thing, be willing to practice returning to mindfulness again and again. It is gentle, self-accepting persistence that reaches the goal (if we can speak of a goal), not pushing, striving, or struggling. Be like the waves of water, which overpower the hard rock by being willing to return again and again and again. This is completely natural. All of us who are not yet full-time Buddhas have moments of forgetfulness. When you find yourself having lapsed again, perhaps for the thousandth time in a day, laugh and smile. As a recovering person, you know a lot about the power of habit energy. Don't let it catch you in frustration and impatience.

Remember that mindfulness is "choiceless awareness"; that is, it is the willingness to be present with *whatever* is going on. This includes being willing to become aware of your forgetfulness and to return again to mindfulness. If you become self-critical or frustrated, you have become too goal oriented about your spiritual practice. Relax. Use humor. Smile. Tune into the fun. Isn't it funny that, while we are already Buddhas, we forget our true nature over and over and over again? Isn't it funny that, if we struggle too hard, we get caught in the very net of suffering we want to escape? These habit energies just need to play themselves out. They are us. If we fight with them, we fight with ourselves and only make them stronger.

In *Opening the Eye of New Awareness* (1999), the Dalai Lama quoted another lama as saying: "Suddenly looking at it, it may seem as if it is impossible for someone like oneself to be able to do these things. However, compounded phenomena [such as human beings] do not remain as they are; they change with conditions. If you do not become discouraged and keep working at it, something that you think could not be produced in a hundred years is one day produced."

Make patience and self-acceptance your main practice. And one day you will realize you have changed. You will see that you have become a more mindful person. You get there, not by trying all at once to attain some perfection, but just by the simple daily things we have been talking about. You get there one mindful breath at a time. Ching-yuan comments in *The Way of Zen*:

Before I had studied Zen for 30 years, I saw mountains as mountains, and waters as waters. When I arrived at a more intimate knowledge, I came to the point where I saw that mountains are not mountains, and waters are not waters. But now that I have got its very substance I am at rest. For it's just that I see mountains once again as mountains, and waters once again as waters.

When you get there, you know it is where you have always been. You know it is your true home.

Recommended Reading

For additional resources, including Internet sites and an updated reading list, visit us at mindfulpsychology.com.

Anonymous. *The Cloud of Unknowing.* Translated by Clifton Walters. Harmondsworth, England: Penguin, 1961.

Charlotte Joko Beck. *Everyday Zen: Love and Work.* San Francisco: HarperSanFrancisco, 1989.

Herbert Benson. M.D. *The Relaxation Response.* New York: Avon, 1975.

Sylvia Boorstein. *It's Easier Than You Think: The Buddhist Way to Happiness.* San Francisco: HarperSanFrancisco, 1997.

Frederick Buechner. *Now and Then.* San Francisco: Harper & Row, 1983.

Joseph Campbell with Bill Moyers. *The Power of Myth.* New York: Doubleday, 1988.

David A. Cooper. *A Heart of Stillness: A Complete Guide to Learning the Art of Meditation.* Woodstock, Vt.: SkyLight Paths Publishing, 1999.

H. H. the Dalai Lama and Howard C. Cutler, M.D. *The Art of Happiness: A Handbook for Living.* New York: Riverhead, 1998.

Catherine de Hueck Doherty. *Poustinia: Christian Spirituality of the East for Western Man.* Notre Dame: Ave Maria Press, 1975.

Ralph Waldo Emerson. *Selected Writings of Ralph Waldo Emerson.* Edited by William Gilman. New York: Signet, 1965.

Mark Epstein, M.D. *Thoughts without a Thinker: Psychotherapy from a Buddhist Perspective.* New York: Basic Books, 1995.

Matthew Fox. *The Reinvention of Work: A New Vision of Livelihood for Our Time.* San Francisco: HarperSanFrancisco, 1994.

Andrew Harvey. *The Way of Passion: A Celebration of Rumi.* Berkeley, Calif.: Frog, Ltd., 1994.

Robert A. Johnson with Jerry M. Ruhl. *Balancing Heaven and Earth.* San Francisco: HarperSanFrancisco, 1998.

Jon Kabat-Zinn. *Full Catastrophe Living: Using the Wisdom of Your Body and Mind to Face Stress, Pain, and Illness.* New York: Delta, 1990.

———. *Wherever You Go, There You Are: Mindfulness Meditation in Everyday Life.* New York: Hyperion, 1994.

Jack Kornfield. *After the Ecstasy, the Laundry: How the Heart Grows Wise on the Spiritual Path.* New York: Bantam, 2000.

Lao Tzu. *The Way of Life According to Lao Tzu.* Translated by Witter Bynner. New York: Capricorn, 1962.

Brother Lawrence. *The Practice of the Presence of God.* Edited by Donald Demaray. New York: Alba House, 1997.

Stephen Levine. *A Gradual Awakening.* New York: Doubleday, 1979.

Thomas Merton. *New Seeds of Contemplation.* New York: New Directions, 1961.

———. *Mystics and Zen Masters.* New York: Dell, 1967.

Thomas Moore. *Care of the Soul.* New York: Harper Perennial, 1992.

———. *The Re-Enchantment of Everyday Life.* New York: Harper Collins, 1996.

———. *Soul Mates: Honoring the Mysteries of Love and Relationship.* New York: HarperCollins, 1994.

Henri J. M. Nouwen. *The Wounded Healer: Ministry in Contemporary Society.* New York: Doubleday, 1972.

Sharon Salzberg. *A Heart As Wide as the World: Living with Mindfulness, Wisdom, and Compassion.* Boston: Shambhala, 1997.

John A. Sanford. *Healing and Wholeness.* New York: Paulist Press, 1977.

Lama Surya Das. *Awakening the Buddha Within: Tibetan Wisdom for the Western World.* New York: Broadway, 1997.

Shunryu Suzuki. *Zen Mind, Beginner's Mind.* New York: Weatherhill, 1970.

Thich Nhat Hanh. *The Miracle of Mindfulness.* Boston: Beacon Press, 1975.

———. *Being Peace.* Berkeley, Calif.: Parallax Press, 1987.

———. *Peace Is Every Step: The Path of Mindfulness in Everyday Life.* New York: Bantam, 1991.

———. *Living Buddha, Living Christ.* New York: Riverhead, 1995.

———. *The Heart of the Buddha's Teaching: Transforming Suffering into Peace, Joy, and Liberation; The Four Noble Truths, The Noble Eightfold Path, and Other Basic Buddhist Teachings.* Berkeley, Calif.: Parallax Press, 1998.

Swami Vivekananda. *Meditation and Its Methods.* Hollywood: Vedanta Press, 1946.

Alan Watts. *The Way of Zen.* New York: Vintage, 1957.

Index